DISCONJUGATE GAZE

By Daniel Rufer

<u>**Dedication**</u>

To my lioness and wife (Kirstin) whose courage, bravery, love, and support could not possibly be captured in this book. For all the maneuvering and strong-arming you did to keep me safe and comfortable. For all the lonely nights you spent at home while I was in the hospital and all the painful conversations you had on my behalf. I am forever indebted as your partner. I love you deeply and forever. This book is for you.

Author's Note

This book is a memoir that I never intended to write. The primary document used in the recreation of the experiences portrayed in this book is an "accomplishments journal" Kirstin kept for me in which we recorded at least one "accomplishment" every day for the first 100 days post-surgery.

The situations portrayed in this book are accurate subject to the notes in my accomplishments journal and my memory. When possible, I sent excerpts of the book to real-life characters for content verification.

The dialogue in this book is accurate to my memory, not to transcription.

The names of all health care professionals have been changed to protect their privacy, but the names of (almost) every non-healthcare character in the book are real.

In an effort to bring awareness to traumatic brain injury and support those individuals and families that experience such life-altering events, 10% of the proceeds from this work will be set aside to benefit research on brain injuries, cavernous malformations, and strokes.

Because I have lost dexterity and significant sensation in my left hand, the vast majority of this work was created using dictation software.

CONTENTS

GREY GOOSE ON THE ROCKS

"Grey Goose on the rocks, small ice, and three olives, please." I turned to my friend Dave, who had already ordered a beer.

"So why are you not at work today?"

"It's a long story. Mind if we wait for the drinks and I'll tell you all about it?"

"No problem. Are you okay?"

"I think so, but remember that thing that I was having with my back?" Dave nodded.
"Well, the doctors aren't exactly sure if the numbness in my foot is caused by my back. I think they're full of shit." Our drinks arrived. "Cheers!" We clicked our glasses, but before I could take a sip my phone rang. "Excuse me a second, I think this is the doctor calling. I have to take this."

"Hi, doc. No, I can't hear you. I'm meeting a friend for a drink. Hold on a second, let me step outside…"

"Hello, Daniel. Can you hear me now?

"Yes, Dr. Adams. I can hear you fine," I said as I crossed the threshold out of the cold, dark, air-conditioned bar to the warm sunny spring air of NYC in April. "Tell me good news," I implored. I should have known something was wrong. Doctors never call you back on the same day of an MRI.

"So, the good news is that you don't have MS." My throat tightened, and I braced for the bad news that inevitably follows a setup like that. "The MRI showed that you have something called a cavernous malformation. We think that's what's causing the numbness on the left side of your body. I've already called the emergency room at the hospital. I need you to go home and pack a bag. You're going to be spending the night."

"Whoa whoa whoa. Are you serious? The numbness is sciatica. You just told me I don't have MS." I paused. "So, what is this cavernous mal *what* thing?"

"I can't fully explain that right now, but we need you to go to the hospital so that you can be observed overnight. You'll be able to meet with a surgeon who will be able to tell you more about your condition."

"Wait, what? A surgeon. A brain surgeon. What are we talking about? My wife just got on a plane to Chicago. I can't go the hospital today. Can I just go on Friday, when she gets back?"

"No, the surgeon I want you to meet is only there tonight. You need to pack a bag and go to the hospital," the doctor said in a stern voice.

"Okay." I paused. "This is a lot to take in on a Wednesday afternoon."

"I know it is, Daniel, but you need to go to the hospital. This doctor knows that you're coming and can assess the situation better than I can. He is the best surgeon for these types of situations."

"You keep calling him a surgeon. Am I going to have brain surgery tonight?" I must have been yelling. The five or six people who were seated at the outdoor tables turned their heads and looked at me. I turned away from the crowd of bystanders and in a lower voice I said, "Do I have time to walk the dog?"

"Yes, but walk the dog, pack a bag, and head to the hospital. I've already called ahead. The receptionist at the emergency room is expecting you and the surgeon knows that you are spending the night."

"Okay, what's the name of this thing again?" She said it one more time, but I couldn't understand it any better this time around. I tapped the phone to end the call and walked back inside the bar.

"Dave." I paused. "I've got to go to the hospital"

"What? What's going on? What did the doctor say?

"The doc said there is something wrong with the MRI report and I have to go in for overnight observation. I'm meeting with a brain surgeon." I paused. "Can you watch my dog? Can you watch Moxie?"

"Sure. Just let me chug this beer first." I must have been outside a little while because his pint was already almost half-finished. He gulped the last eight ounces, I threw a twenty on the bar, and we walked back to my apartment.

EMERGENCY ROOM SLUMBER PARTY

What does one pack for an overnight stay at a hospital? It's not like I was having a baby and planned a "go bag." I was the recipient of a phone call from a doctor at approximately 5:00 p.m. and was told in no uncertain terms that I needed to get to the emergency room immediately to stay overnight for observation. Did I need extra underwear? Did I need socks? Would they be providing me with a toothbrush and toothpaste? What kind of book should one bring while waiting for terrible news under fluorescent lights?

I don't think I actually had any of those thoughts; I simply grabbed a gym bag, threw in a pair of shorts, a t-shirt, an extra pair of underwear, and ran out of the apartment door, leaving Dave to care for my one-year-old morkie named Moxie. Things happened very quickly that day and I don't remember much of any of the phone conversations I had in the taxi on the way to the hospital, but I do know that I called my wife first, my parents second, and my boss third. Unfortunately, my wife was traveling for work and, as I would learn later, got my voicemail after landing in Detroit as part of a planned layover for her flight to Chicago. To say that leaving a voicemail for my wife explaining that I was headed towards the emergency room for a brain-related condition was beyond my standard greeting communique is an understatement. I don't know exactly what I said, but knowing myself it probably undersold the seriousness of the situation and went something like this: "Hey honey, it's me. I hope your flight is going well. So, I'm on my way to the hospital.

It's probably not a big deal, but the doctor didn't like something about my MRI and wants me to meet with a brain surgeon. Anyway, I love you and call me when you get to your hotel room in Chicago." My wife and I are total opposites. Having just received life-altering news, I'm quite sure that I left a very level-headed just-the-facts-style message that drove her insane. Luckily, she saw through all of that and begged, pleaded, and New-York-style screamed her way to a return ticket and got to the hospital around midnight.

My second phone call was to my parents, or more specifically to my mother. It was, after all, April 15th, 2015. April 15th is the most stressful day in the calendar year because April 15th is Tax Day, and my father is an accountant. Not that phoning him ever occurred to me, but I also knew that he was busy. My mother actually knew that I had gone for the MRI earlier that day, so she was on guard as soon as I called her. I don't think I had to say much to her on the phone before she asked me, "Which hospital?"

"You don't have to come. I'm just here for observation. It's probably nothing." That's most likely what I said in the phone call, when in fact I knew enough to know that even if this visit was not catastrophic, it was something big and I was scared.

"Okay, well what time is Kirstin getting there?" she asked, referring to my wife.

"I couldn't get in touch with her; she's on a flight to Chicago for work"

"We're coming. See you in thirty minutes." And she hung up the phone.

My third and final phone call ended almost as I got to the hospital. It was to my boss, Hugo. I didn't get him either, but I left a voicemail saying that the doctors wanted me to take it easy for another day. I had told him that I was seeing a back specialist as my reason for not being at work earlier in the day, and that I'd call him the next night. I don't remember hearing back from him, so he must have taken that news in stride. But still it must have been annoying for me to call out sick two days in a row. In education, calling in sick was always viewed as a sign of weakness. You never did it unless you had to because you were letting the team down. Perhaps he didn't call me back because he knew something was wrong. Or perhaps he didn't call me back for another reason. I don't know, but I was sure glad not be answering phone calls on that day.

In any event, as the taxi pulled up to the emergency room I remember thinking that I didn't belong... that this was all over some exaggerated or poorly-read MRI. It felt like a mistake walking into that emergency room and much of me wanted to head back home, but I didn't. Perhaps I didn't leave because it wasn't an ER like on TV. There weren't gunshot victims bleeding out on gurneys and family members screaming at nurses for information. In fact, it was quite the opposite. People were waiting patiently to be called, as if they were waiting at a deli counter for some sliced meats rather than waiting to be treated for internal bleeding or a broken bone. It was very civilized, too civilized. A kind young woman in regular professional clothes asked in a department-store-kind-of-way "Can I help you?" It occurred to me that she was some sort of upper east side emergency room "greeter."

I replied "I'm not sure. My doctor told me to come here and that you would be expecting me. I don't really know what--"

"What is your doctor's name?

"Adams. I cannot remember her first name."

She typed something into a computer, looked up, and said, "Daniel."

"Yes, that's me. Does it say why I'm here?"

"I'm sorry, I really don't have that information, but if you follow me, this nurse will check you in." Everyone was so calm. It was as if I was being shown to my rental car rather than my altered future. I was alone and terrified when I sat down in a metal chair with plastic blue upholstery.

"Is there anyone coming to meet you?" the emergency

room flight attendant asked me.

"My parents," I said, feeling a little ashamed to admit that I was still a momma's boy at age 34. "My wife is away on business," I sheepishly added in the hopes of regaining some adulthood in her eyes, but she was gone.

NO URGENCY IN THE EMERGENCY ROOM

This emergency room was devoid of emergencies. Not that that was a bad thing, but things at an Upper East Side emergency room move at a deliberate pace. And even though I was there with a serious condition, of which I currently knew nothing, I was not in an emergency, per se. I would later come to find out that I was simply in the emergency room because that is where the experts were.

Once the receptionist left, a nurse came by to take my temperature and other vital signs. Everything was normal and I again asked, "Do you know why I'm here?" Like the emergency room greeter before her, this woman had no answer for me. She affixed an ID label to a bracelet with my name, age, and morphine allergy printed on it and kindly pointed me back to the waiting area. At this point my parents arrived.

"Hi honey. What's going on? Are you okay?"

"I'm fine. I don't know why I'm here and nobody has an answer for me."

"Did they say how long you are going to be here?

"No."

"Did they say who you are here to see?"

"No."

"Are you being admitted?"

"I don't know." I didn't know the answers to any of these questions and wouldn't know the answers to any of them for many more hours to come. The emergency room waiting area was essentially the first waiting area of this visit. It took about an hour, but they finally took me back to the actual emergency room, where I waited at least another hour to talk to anyone other than a nurse. No new tests, no new information, just waiting

Not that waiting in an emergency room is without entertainment. Depending on what time and where you are waiting, an emergency room can be quite entertaining. My first suite-mate in the emergency room proper was a septuagenarian woman named Gertie. From the moment of her arrival she was mumbling things to herself in (I think) Yiddish. Though I could not understand her, from her tone and body language she did not appear happy. After the second time she tried to leave the emergency room, I asked the nurse why she was here.

"Oh, that's Gertie. She's in here about once a week. She forgets to eat or drink every couple of days. Then she gets dehydrated and ends up here." A simple explanation for a complicated problem.

Gertie continued to mumble to herself and pull the curtain back while looking for an escape route. At some point Gertie broke from her Yiddish mumblings and looked straight at me and said, "Blue Martians." My time with Gertie wasn't restful but at least it was entertaining. For those two or three hours I definitely was more focused on her mumblings and trying to decipher when I was going to meet the blue Martians than on thinking about my own future.

It was a relatively quiet night by emergency room standards. There was no "code blue" calls and I never once saw the defibrillator machine go racing by. The beds were not at full occupancy and most of the time the nurses had time to chat with each other at the central desk. This is not a bad thing, but when you check in to a hospital with an unknown illness at 6:00 p.m. and by 11:00 p.m. you still haven't seen a doctor, your nerves are not exactly calmed by the monotony of a routine emergency room shift.

The first doctor that I did see was a piece of shit. While he might have been as old as 26, he looked 16 and probably

Daniel Rufer

only needed to shave once every three days. "Mr. Ruffer," he said without looking up from his chart. He nailed the double threat of terrible bedside manner coupled with the mispronunciation of my last name. The second sentence from the prick neurosurgery resident was, "It doesn't look like you need brain surgery tonight." I didn't know brain surgery was on the table, so his phrasing, delivery, and overall douchebaggery was not comforting. Still without looking up from his chart, he continued. "The cavernous malformation appears to have stabilized, but we're going to want to keep you here overnight. Have you seen Dr. Ross yet?"

"Who?"

"Dr. Ross. He's the neurosurgeon on call tonight."

"Um, no. So, you're not the guy I'm here to see."

"No, I'm a resident."

"Great, thanks. Could you find the nurse for me?"

"Nurse!" he bellowed into the hallway. "Do you have any questions for me?" He finally looked up.

"For you... Nope."

MOVING ON UP

It couldn't have been more than 30 minutes later that my mother got a text from Kirstin saying that she was on her way back from the airport. I remember seeing her in the hallway between the waiting room and the emergency room with her rolling suitcase dragging behind her. I had held it together up until this point, but as soon as I saw my wife I started to cry.

I left my bed and walked toward her. She hugged me deeply for about ten seconds before asking, "What's going on, honey? I got your message and talked to your mom, but what is happening?"

"I still don't know, but the doctor was talking about brain surgery." She looked me in the eyes and began sobbing audibly. Her chest heaved with each sniffle. We stood there hugging, looking over each other's shoulder, for what felt like five minutes. When my mother approached us carrying bottled water from the cafeteria, I broke away from my wife's embrace, wiped my eyes and nose, and tried to compose myself. My mother simply handed us the two bottles, hugged Kirstin, and walked away. We waited in the corridor for another minute or so before returning to the emergency room stall.

DR. MCDREAMY

My parents left us around 1 a.m. The doctors moved me upstairs to the neurology ward around 2:00 a.m. On the 6th floor, the nurses explained to me that the doctor I was supposed to see had already gone home, but that he would check in with me upon arrival tomorrow morning. When that would be exactly they could not tell me, but it would probably be before noon. Even though it was 2:00 a.m. and I hadn't had a coffee for at least 10 hours, I was wide awake. There are few things less common than being told you are a candidate for brain surgery with no follow-up whatsoever and then having leads attached to your hairy chest at 2:00 in the morning. I asked one of the nurses for something to help me sleep. They refused, but eventually I fell asleep on my own and I was able to get a solid four hours that night. I slept in a bed and my wife slept on a battered blue plastic armchair.

Around 7:00 a.m., the lights came on and a nurse entered the room to wake us up. "The doctor is in the hospital and will be coming by shortly," she said with a smile as she fluffed my pillow. Minutes after the morning sun had begun to fill our south-facing room, Dr. Ross crossed the threshold of the doorway. He was flanked by four interns in white coats who in this lighting, and in my tired state, reminded me of softly lit doves. "Daniel?" he asked.

"Yes. This is my wife--"

"Kirstin," she said, leaning over my body from the left side of the hospital bed with an outstretched hand and a mile-wide smile. It was a little ridiculous to see your wife fawning over a doctor she had never met while her husband lay in a hospital bed awaiting life-altering news, but I also struggled not to giggle. To put it in mildly, he was tall, dark, and handsome. To put it less mildly, he was stupid hot. He was wearing a custom-tailored blue-pattern suit, matching blue tie, and white pocket square. I would later learn that he was exactly my age, but the confidence and posture of this man gave him an authority over the room that made me feel like a child.

"Hello, Mrs. Rufer," he said, offering his hand with a smile that I could feel made my wife's knees buckle.

"It's Bunton," she said coyly.

"Okay," I interjected, trying to redirect the interaction to my pending health crisis and away from my wife's newest crush. "What can you tell me, doctor? Why am I here?"

"Mr. Rufer, you have a cavernous malformation located just to the right of your brainstem." One of the white coats took out an MRI scan and placed it in the doctor's hand. "You can see it right here. It's the dark spot on the scan." I couldn't decipher one bit of the scan from any other; it looked like a bowl of pasta surrounded with some flattened meatballs, but I nodded. "The cavernous malformation is a cluster of blood vessels that some-times can get twisted and rupture with a bleed. That's what happened with your malformation and that's what is causing the numbness in your foot."

"Are you sure? Isn't this just an issue with my back?"

"I don't think so. The good news is your cavernous mal-formation is very small. And most of the time a rupture is a one-time thing that resolves itself on its own. I imagine that in a couple of weeks sensation will return to your leg and you'll be able to live a normal, healthy life."

I asked the obvious question: "What if the numbness doesn't go away or gets worse?"

"Well, let's hope it doesn't come to that." He paused. "Your cav-mal is in a very eloquent place. I don't know if you remember your high school biology, but the brainstem controls many important functions throughout the body, including lung function. Because the cav-mal is on the right side of your brain-stem you have numbness in the left side of your body. There are many nerves that run into and out of the brain stem. Because this is such an important area of the brain, surgery is not really an option. And I would be wary of any neurologist that told you differently. Even if the numbness doesn't resolve itself, the risks of a surgery to this particular area of the brain are vast, so surgery should not be considered lightly."

My wife interjected: "So, what can we do to help him heal?"

"As I said earlier, this situation will likely resolve itself on its own, but if it doesn't we can schedule another MRI and discuss your options in my office. I have to continue on my rounds, but Kimberly will walk you through my recommendation and give you all my information." And with that, he flashed another golden smile, shook my hand, said, "take care" and was gone.

Kimberly was one of the white coats with which he had arrived. We would later find out that she was a nurse practitioner who worked with Dr. Ross. She sat on the edge of the bed and begin to address the two of us in a calming voice. The rest of his entourage had left the room and it was just Kimberly, myself, and Kirstin. "Dr. Ross is recommending seven to ten days of rest. No work. No exercise. And nothing that would get your heart rate up. That also includes no drinking, no drugs, no alcohol, and no sex."

"No sex!" I responded with exasperation. "You know we are newlyweds, right?"

She smiled a little. "This is serious. Anything that raises your heart rate could trigger another bleed, but the longer you go without another bleed the less likely it is to recur. So, he is recommending two weeks off from work. What do you do for a living? Can you do that?"

"Not really," I said. "I'm a teacher. I've already missed parent conference day yesterday and there are only so many weeks left in the school year--"

My wife cut me off: "He'll do it."

"How about ten days? Through the following Sunday." It

was now Thursday morning.

"Okay, but you really need to take it easy until then. Take this card. Call us if anything comes up and make an appointment for that Monday. He'll want to see you before you can go back to work."

"So, can we go home now?"

"I'll get somebody working on your discharge papers and call in a nurse to remove the EEG leads." We were home an hour later.

NOW WHAT?

It was late morning by the time we got home. The first thing I did was address the painful bald patches throughout my hairy chest. It was like that gruesome scene in *The 40-Year-Old Virgin*, complete with searing pain and small droplets of blood. Despite 20 minutes of vigorous scrubbing in the shower with multiple soap canisters I was unable to remove all of the adhesive, so I spent most of the rest of the afternoon with no shirt on. The rectangular bald patches on my otherwise hairy chest looked like an abstract painting.

'Now what?" I asked my wife. "I'm not very good at sitting around."

"Now we watch Netflix and ignore what just happened"," she mused.

The advent of digital streaming on Netflix is the greatest comfort to the couch-bound mid-thirties male. Despite growing up in the age of television, the old adage "100 channels and nothin' on," still held true for late morning and early afternoon television. Sportscenter was stale at that point, but with Netflix, *Seinfeld*, *30 Rock*, and *Always Sunny* were my comfort in a time of needed distraction.

I'm sure there were some tears, hugs, and difficult conversations in the 10 days I spent on bedrest. But what I remember most is boredom, Netflix streaming, and deliveries by Seamless.

RETURN TO WORK

Twelve days after my overnight in the hospital, I was cleared to return to work. On the Thirteenth day, a Tuesday, I did just that. The first couple of days back were, as one might imagine, were difficult. They weren't difficult because of the high-energy kids or my own sense of impending doom, they were difficult because I was lying to everyone. The greetings I got from students usually went like this:

"Hey, Mr. Rufer. Glad to see you back, what happened?"

"Hey, Mr. Rufer. The sub really sucked while you were out. Don't ever leave again. Are you okay?"

"Hey, Mr. Rufer. You look totally fine; are you scamming the school?"

My answer was always the same. It was the same in a robotic sort of way that usually allows me to tell when children are lying to me about something. Yet, none of them ever called me out on the lie. Maybe I'm really good at lying, or may they were really bad at detecting it. Whatever the case, my story always went like this:

"Thanks for asking, student X. I tweaked my back lifting weights. The doctor made me stay in bed for ten days. It was really boring, but at least I had Netflix." That usually satisfies them. With adults, my story was a bit more elaborate. Bigger people require bigger lies, or at least more detailed lies. The kids never asked follow-up questions. Adults almost always did. Either they or a friend had gone through some kind of back injury, so I had to give more details: "I tweaked my L4 and L5 vertebrae. The doctor doesn't think I need surgery, but I have to take it easy for a while and get reevaluated over the summer."

For most that was sufficient, but for some adults it wasn't. Usually, the older colleagues would ask me:

"Who is your doctor?"

"What hospital is he affiliated with?"

"My nephew is a radiologist, do you want me to get him to look at it?"

On day one, these questions really threw me for a loop, but I went home that night and did some research on back surgeons. Luckily for me, but unluckily for my father, he had back surgery two years prior, so I eventually made myself his fake patient. "I'm working with Dr. Such-and-such at hospital X. I'm comfortable working with him for now, but if I need a second opinion, I'll definitely call you."

After a couple of days, the questions about my absence slowed to a manageable level and I got back to doing what I did best: teaching algebra and yelling at kids who are out of dress code. As a teacher, the enforcement of school rules is not about a visible show of force like standing in the hall asking a child to tuck in their shirt like you might have seen in the movies. The key is the element of surprise. Being a grade dean, my teaching load was half that of a normal teacher, and I spent most of the rest of my time walking the hallways, opening classroom doors and confiscating hats. Or waiting in a bathroom stall for twenty minutes of silence only to burst out and confiscate four cell phones of texting teenage boys. It's more work than standing in one place at classes change, but guerrilla-style enforcement is the only way to keep students on edge about rules violations.

DO YOU HEAR THAT RINGING?

Other than slight numbness in my left foot and leg, the month of May was fairly normal. I woke up at 6:30, showered, applied leave-in conditioner to my hair, went to work, taught something about quadratic functions, confiscated a few phones, and went to the gym. Rinse and repeat. Then, on the Wednesday following Memorial Day, something changed that made my situation far more serious. I started to experience a ringing in my left ear. I know it was on a Wednesday because I was teaching a course called Urban Studies, which I only teach on Wednesdays. I may have woken up with the ringing, but I only noticed it when a latecomer slammed the door upon entering the classroom. I figured it was something related to sinus pressure from allergies and ignored it as best I could while I got the lesson underway. About 15 minutes into the class I remember asking a child quietly at her desk if she also heard the ringing. When she said no, my heart sank and I figuratively held my breath until lunchtime, when I could call my doctor.

As soon as class ended, I retreated to my office and called my general practitioner. I left a message for her explaining the ringing in my left ear and asking what I should do and if it was related to the cavernous malformation. Kindly, I got a return phone call from my doctor urging me not to worry and to make an appointment with an ear, nose and throat (ENT) Doctor as soon as possible. When I scheduled an appointment for first thing Friday morning, I felt a little better.

But when I woke up the next morning with a tingling sensation in my left thumb, I felt a lot worse.

DOCTORS, DOCTORS, AND MORE DOCTORS

On that Friday morning I visited with the ENT, Dr. Stevenson.

"The ringing I hear can best be described as a low-pitched buzzing sound that you might hear after a television had been turned off. It's worse on the street or on the train."

"Do you hear it when a room is completely quiet?"

"Hold on a sec," I said and held up my finger and counted to five. "No, but the buzzing kind of trails off like a tuning fork." I paused. "It's back now."

"Okay, let me examine your ears, then your nose, and then your throat. That's why they call me an ENT," he said with a smile and a chuckle. I think it was supposed to be a joke, but I was in no laughing mood. He poked one of those ear microscope things in each ear lightly, then jammed the same one up my nose roughly, before asking me to say "ahh" and turning away to discard the disposable plastic scope cover. "I see a little swelling in the sinus cavity, but nothing too serious. I'm going to start you on a course of antibiotics and see if that clears things up."

"So, have you spoken to Dr. Adams, because I have this cavernous malformation thing and--"

"Yes. I know. I got a message from her yesterday. We went to medical school together, you know," he said, as if their familiarity would lighten the mood. "It's possible that the cav-mal could be causing the tinnitus in your ear, but it's worth pursuing the antibiotics first before ordering any other tests." The doctor ripped the prescription off the pad and handed it to me.

"Thank you," I said sheepishly, placing the prescription in my pocket. He was correct that it was the prudent course of action, but it didn't make me feel any better. I was worried about the tinnitus, but I was even more worried about the numbness on the left side of my body, which had now partially engulfed my entire left leg and was spreading from my thumb to the lower part of my wrist and hand. Luckily, I only taught one class on Fridays, so I hopped on the subway downtown to deliver an uninspiring lesson on the unit circle.

The following week the month of June began, and with it a slew of additional doctor's appointments. On Tuesday I met with the back doctor whom I had used as part of my false narrative at school. It was a long shot, but I had convinced this doctor, my father's doctor, to examine me for sciatica or anything else that could cause the numbness on the left side of my body. By the time I had all the tests done for this appointment the numbness has spread in such a way that the outcome was not a surprise. I waited in his office for about an hour in a paper gown only for him to come in and tell me in a few words that there was nothing wrong with my back. Under most circumstances that would be great news, but I hoping for damage to my spine that could explain the other issues I was having with my body rather than a vascular anomaly pressing on my brain stem.

By Wednesday of that week the numbness had spread from the top of my ear to the base of my neck on the left side of my body. It wasn't complete numbness, but it felt different to the touch. The numbness in my left foot and my left hand had gotten worse as well. The feeling that can best describe it is what you feel right after smacking your funny bone on the side of a table. Except that that feeling goes away and this one never did.

By Thursday, even though I appeared calm at work, I was in full freak-out mode. I was able to secure an appointment on Friday at noon with the original neurologist, Dr. Adams. It was clear to me that something had gone wrong or dramatically progressed. I went to work on Friday and cut out around noon.

I phoned Kirstin on the train to the doctor while hyperventilating and thinking I was going to die. The doctor conceded that it was necessary to take another MRI and pulled some strings to get us in the next evening at 8:00 p.m. Not the sexiest of Saturday night activities, but very necessary.

BACK TO DR. ROSS AND THE PENULTIMATE DAY OF SCHOOL

I had an appointment to meet with Dr. Ross at 3:30 p.m. on Monday, June 15th. It was the last full day of classes for the 2014-2015 school year. My wife met me at the doctor's office, and thankfully we didn't have to wait long. Once we got called back to the office I don't think we were talking to each other at all.

In walked Dr. Ross, this time in scrubs. He didn't have a trail of interns following him, just his trusty nurse practitioner Kimberly. This time around there was less of an aura around him and there was far less giggling on the part of my wife.

"Okay, Daniel. Let's start with what we know." He pulled up a set of images on the computer. He scrolled through the file using his index finger over the mouse and stopped on a particular image. "Do you see that dark area?" This time I did. "That's the cavernous malformation." He opened a second file, and scrolled to the corresponding image on the MRI from six weeks ago. "This is that same slice of the MRI from the original scan, back in April." I didn't see anything. Then he pointed using his pen and I could make out a dark circle about the size of a dime. "if you look at the image on the right from last Saturday, you can see that the malformation has gotten significantly larger." I could see that what had gone from the size of a dime was now about the size of a quarter.

"So, you think that's what's causing the extra numbness?"

"Yes."

"And the ringing in my ear?"

"Yes."

"So, what do we do? You previously said that surgery was not an option you would recommend."

"I did and it wasn't, but given the growth of the cav-mal, we should at least discuss surgery." Kirstin squeezed my hand.

"Are you suggesting that I have brain surgery? Isn't that risky?"

"It is and I'm not suggesting anything. I'm actually quite torn on your specific case." Not what you expect to hear from a surgeon. "I presented your case to my colleagues on the surgical board and five out of nine recommended surgery. The other four recommended waiting." I squeezed back.

"What do you think?"

"I'm not sure. Let me give you all the facts and then you two can make the decision. Sometimes I recommend surgery right away, but other times it's more complicated. Here's why. Remember that I described the location of the cavernous malformation as being eloquent." I nodded. He pointed his pen at the MRI image once again. "Well, the cav-mal you have is resting just to the right of the brain stem. The brain stem is essentially the connection between your brain and the rest of your body. When the cav-mal ruptured the first time it bled to the left, damaging the peripheral nerves to the left side of your body. But those aren't the only nerves that run through this small area. In fact, the nerves that control movement to your right eye and the right side of your face are also just on the edge of the cav-mal. More importantly, there are nerves that control involuntary muscles like your lungs and the ability to swallow that also operate in this area. So, the problem is not getting rid of the cav-mal, the problem is getting to it." He paused and looked back towards Kirstin and me. "In order to remove the cav-mal, which I'm confident I can do, I need to cut through some existing cranial nerves that are thus far undamaged. I'd have to cut through cranial nerves 6 and 7. Those control movement to the right side of your face and to your right eye. You would lose movement on the right side of your face and be left with a disconjugate gaze. In essence you would have double vision." Kirstin pulled her hand away to dab her eye and I noticed how sweaty my left hand had become. My right hand (also sweaty) was gripping the tissue paper of the exam table.

"So, what would happen with the numbness to the left side of my body?"

"If all goes well, it should not get worse and may even abate. The 'buy-in,'" he said, using air quotes, "is the loss of facial movement and the disconjugate gaze."

"How big of a deal is this disconjugate gaze?

"It's a big deal, but it is something you could live with and be successful with. There are some surgeries that could help correct these issues, but they are unlikely to be perfect. Of course, I need to mention that this is brain surgery, and the risks are many. We run the risk of losing lung function and your being connected to a breathing machine. You also run the risk of needing a feeding tube. And death is always a possibility with brain surgery."

"How significant are these complications?" my wife asked.

"I don't expect any of those outcomes," said the doctor confidently, but compassionately.

"Could you give us a percentage?"

"Less than 10%" said the doctor hedging his advice. "The main concern is the facial paralysis and the disconjugate gaze." I could tell he was trying to elicit his best bedside manner. I looked at my wife. We both had red eyes.

As I reached for her hand I asked, "And if we opt to not have surgery?"

"We monitor you and hope that there are no more bleeds."

"But if it bleeds again, I could have all of these problems anyway, right?" I asked. The doctor nodded. Kirstin looked at me and I think we both knew what has to be done at that moment.

"If we decide to have this done, how quickly would we have to act on this?"

"Well, this is not urgent," said the man whose head was not killing him from the inside out. "I'd have to check my calendar" he said, looking at the nurse, "but, if you elect to have surgery, I would think we should do it sooner rather than later."

My wife interjected: "So, we are going on our honeymoon next Friday--"

"Oh jeez," said the surgeon in a way that you could tell he was trying to hold that comment in but had failed.

Kirstin continued: "Could we still go on that if we wanted to?"

"Yes, you can go. Flying is not an issue. Where are you going?" he asked, sounding interested in our social calendar.

"Italy," my wife proclaimed.

"Well, at least you're not in the middle of Africa. You can get medical attention if you need it in Italy. Just travel with your MRI images." I think Kirstin was still hopeful we could make the trip, but I knew I couldn't enjoy a vacation knowing that my body could kill me from within at any moment. "You guys have a lot to talk about. Kimberly will give you my contact information, and please call me with any questions." He extended his hand to me first.

"Any restrictions in the meantime?"

"No, not for right now." He extended his hand to my wife.

"So, we can still roll at the rave in Central Park this weekend." She looked at me while shaking his hand. "That's good news, Danny."

Dr. Ross turned back as if he had swallowed a piece of candy: "I wouldn't recommend that."

"She's joking" I said, and he forced a smile, but I don't think he totally believed me.

Daniel Rufer

As he exited the room, the nurse said, "I thought it was funny." She gave us his card once again and left us in the room to collect ourselves. We collapsed in each other's arms for what seemed like an hour, and we both cried.

END OF (SCHOOL) DAYS

The final day of school at Grace Church School is not graduation, it's something called the closing exercises. After checking in with their advisors, the students head over to the church on 10th Street and Broadway. For this ceremony, the children fill the middle pews. Non-advising faculty and family members fill in the outside. Since most families don't attend and each grade has about 70 students in it, there were about 400 people gathered in the church that morning to celebrate the end of the school year.

Along with the other high school administrators, I sat on the stage facing the students and waiting to give my end-of-year notes. Never one for sentimental feelings, I wrote a speech that I called my SSR. SSR stand for student self-reflection. We ask our students to write the reflections twice a year as a way of getting them to think critically about their academic performance. And they hate this activity.

As 9th grade dean, I had the distinct pleasure (not really) of reading the thoughts of all 74 9th grade students, checking them for spelling and grammatical errors (of which there were many) before they could be published alongside their report card. The perfunctory nature of these children's writings was so comical that I decided to punk them with a self-reflection of my own written with the intonation and vocabulary of a 9th grader. Enjoy:

Overall, I think I did a pretty good job in my first year as a dean at

Grace Church High School. I think I planned a pretty good retreat to start the year and my "spontaneous act of kindness" hot chocolate party seemed to go over pretty well. One thing I would like to improve upon is becoming more approachable. One time this year, there was a birthday party held in my office and I wasn't even invited. Maybe I need to smile more. One thing I think I did well was spot gum-chewers in chapel and assemblies. At the last Chapel only one 9th grader even tried to chew gum and I was able to catch her before the ceremony started. I think I made a real positive impact on the gum-chewing culture of Grace Church School.

In terms of the way I feel, I am very proud of the class of 2018. This year's 9th grade overcame some very real issues both at home and at school. I am most proud of the way the 9th graders opened up to talk about their issue with teachers, counselors, peers, and with me. I think they know, as all GCS students should know, you don't have to go through tough times alone. With specific regard to my 9th graders, I am proud of the way they overcame what life threw at them to end the year on a high note, with both responsibility and dignity. I will enjoy the summer, but I can't wait to get started on the next school year.

Class of 2018, you have met or exceeded the academic requirements for the 9th Grade year of the Grace Church School, High School Division. It is my pleasure to present you to the faculty as the new Sophomore class of Grace Church School.

I got rave reviews for my speech. In an otherwise sentimental ceremony, I provided a sarcastic reprieve from serious thought. I was happy to deliver the speech both for them and for myself. As I left the stage that afternoon, I couldn't help but think that if I were to die over the summer, at least I went out with a bang.

GETTING MY AFFAIRS IN ORDER

It was either later that night or the next morning that we decided to go ahead with the surgery. Thursday, June 25th, 2015 was the day that we set for my cavernous malformation extraction, and it only gave me about one week to get my affairs in order. Being only 35 and married for approximately six months, I had not thought much about my financial situation for the future. But over the next seven days I found every investment account, no matter how small, and registered my wife as the beneficiary. I also employed a lawyer to create a will and a give power of attorney to my wife. I scheduled two surgical consultations with other top neurosurgeons in the area. Both agreed that surgery was the best option.

THE NIGHT BEFORE

The night before my surgery, my wife and I went to dinner at the restaurant where we had our first date. It was a bistro-style restaurant on the Upper West Side of Manhattan that featured pictures of dogs on all of the walls. In fact, there was a picture of Moxie in the back room and one of Lola, our deceased long-haired Chihuahua, by the bathroom entrance.

On the way to the restaurant, I made a phone call to the head of school. I did not expect him to pick up the phone for a strange number at 6:45 on a weekday after school had ended, but he did. I guess he had my number in his phone because he knew who I was immediately

"Hey Dan, how's it going?

"Well, uh, it's going okay. The reason why I'm calling you is to let you know that I'm having surgery tomorrow."

"Okay..."

"It's brain surgery." I paused. "As it turns out, that back thing that kept me out of work in April wasn't a back thing at all, it was a tumor." Technically, it wasn't a tumor, but now was not the time to split hairs. "In any event, I've seen multiple specialists, and we've decided to have surgery tomorrow to remove the tumor."

"Whoa, that's what you call big time surgery," he said, as if the two of us were splitting a beer in a pub.

"Yeah, it's pretty serious. The surgery should be about five hours. My wife has your phone number and will give you a call when I'm on the other side. Poor choice of words. But she will call you when I'm in recovery." I paused. "Mr. Davison, I'm calling you because nobody at work besides Lindsey knows about this. I'd like to keep it that way."

"Not a problem, Dan. I look forward to seeing you later this summer."

"Thank you, sir." I said and ended the phone call. I turned to my wife. "Okay, there's nothing left to do now except to eat dinner, walk the dog, and go to sleep."

"I don't want to do this," my wife said with tears welling in her eyes. "I don't want you to do this."

"Everything is going to be fine. I'm going to be fine."

"But what if it's not?" she said. "What if something happens to you in surgery and I have to make one of those decisions?" she said, referring to the health care proxy I'd made her sign the day before. "I can't do that. I can't make that kind of decision. I don't want you to do this." We stopped walking and embraced.

"I'm going to be fine. You're going to be fine. Everything is going to be fine. This doctor is excellent. The hospital is excellent. I'll be up and about in about in a week, you'll see. Everything is going to be fine." I must admit that I had my doubts about the surgery as well, but I figured if it went poorly I would simply die. I didn't much consider the possibility of being maintained on life support. Selfishly, I figured I would go in for the surgery and either I would make it out or I wouldn't. And I had (sort of) made peace with that.

When we arrived at the restaurant, we were seated at a two-top. I asked Kirstin, "What would make you feel better about tomorrow? What else can we do for you? Your parents will be there. My parents will be there. Your sister is coming in from North Carolina. I'll be knocked out for several hours, so what can we do to make this better for you?"

"I don't know," she said. "I don't want you to do this." Our drinks arrived. She had a glass of wine. I had a seltzer with a lime slice. "Maybe if we set some goals together. Maybe we can set some goals for after your surgery?"

"Like what? I don't understand."

"Things that we're going to do together after the surgery.

Like, go to the beach. Take Moxie to the dog park. Or buy your wife an anniversary necklace."

I chuckled. "Okay, let me think."

"The surgery is on June 25th. When do you want to go to the beach?"

"Let's say you and I will swim the ocean on my birthday, August 6th."

"Okay, that's a good one. Now I'd like to select one for me. I'd like to have a hot dog and a beer on July 4th."

"Great." She laughed. "You can get food poisoning to celebrate your good health. Let's add something that's more physical. What would be a good goal for you in terms of playing golf?"

"How about Labor Day?"

"Okay, so we've got three good goals. One, a hot dog on July 4th." Her face puckered

"And a beer," I interjected.

"One, just the hot dog," Kirstin looked at me sternly. "Two, swim the ocean on August 6th. Three, play golf on Labor Day. So, hot dog, swim the ocean, play golf. Those are three good goals. Will you promise that you will do all of these things?"

I smiled at her. "I promise."

After dinner we walked home together hand-in-hand. We walked the dog together that night as well. I felt good about our plan. I liked Kirstin's suggestion of keeping goals at the forefront of our thoughts. I felt close to her, closer than I think I had felt even at our wedding. That closeness was comforting in what had otherwise been a very stressful couple of weeks. I felt calm getting into bed that night. But that calm dissipated quickly once the lights went out. Kirstin was the first to fall asleep, and even though we were nestled together with the dog in the bed, I was more scared than I had been this entire time. I tried to put it out of mind. I tried to think of the goals we were going to accomplish with the rest of our summer, but the longer I stayed awake the more anxious I became. At 1:00 a.m., I woke Kirstin up.

"What's wrong, baby?" she asked in a tired and confused voice.

"I don't want to die," I said, pulling her closer. "I don't want to die. I don't want to die." I repeated it again and again. "I thought I was okay with everything. I thought I had made peace with everything, but I don't want to die. I want to be there for you and our unborn kids. I want to be with you. I don't want to die."

"You're not going to die." She turned over to face me and rubbed my back. It was her turm to comfort me. "You've got the best doctor in the world and you're going to be fine. You're going to be fine," she repeated. The dog jumped up in between us and licked my tears away. "You're going to be fine. Just keep repeating the goals. If you can do that you will be fine and I'll know you are fine."

"Hot dog, ocean, golf," I said.

"Hot dog, ocean, golf," she repeated.

"Hot dog, ocean, golf," we said together, and we repeated it several more times until we both drifted off to sleep.

THE DAY OF

Thursday, June 25th, 2015 was just like any other day except that I woke up at 4:45 in the morning and took a cab to the Upper East Side for brain surgery. The sun was still rising over the East River as we entered the hospital's automated revolving door. The lobby of the hospital at 5:30 in the morning was a little different than what I would come to know of the hospital during normal business hours. There was only one officer at the security desk, the gift store was closed, and there were no other people anywhere in eyesight or earshot. The sounds of our footsteps echoed off the marble floors and through the empty corridors. Kirstin and I zigzagged our way through the maze of hallways that connected the hospital's many buildings to the "H" elevator bank. We rode to the third floor, turned right, and checked in with the nurse at the "pre-op" desk. She looked up my name, said, "Right this way Daniel," and walked us to one of four curtain-protected eight-foot-by-eight-foot rooms. As I sat down on the blue-green reclining chair she said, "Put this on and fill these out. I'll be back in a few minutes to take your vitals." The gravity of the day began to sink in as she left us alone.

As soon as the curtains closed, Kirstin let the tears fall from her eyes and said, "I don't want to do this," struggling to catch her breath.

"I... We have to do this" I said as I squeezed her hand. "Everything is going to be fine. Hot dog, ocean, golf," I said.

"Hot dog, ocean, golf," she repeated, and hugged me around the neck.

After a short embrace I said to her, "Everything is going to be fine. I love you," and turned my intention to the forms.

Mercifully, there were not that many to fill out. I'm guessing that for brain surgery they have to do so much background that a write-up from the patient on the morning of is not all that important. I signed all the requisite waivers, checked the required boxes, and initialed where asked. Then we waited. We waited in silence, holding hands, trying to find strength in the other's gaze.

After what felt like hours, but was probably only a few minutes, Dr. Ross pulled back the curtain and entered the room looking rested and vigorous, like somebody who had just showered after a quick workout. Maybe he had done just that. It was comforting to see him so cool, confident, and alert as we were melting down. This man was somehow just as attractive wearing scrubs that cost a combined $5 as he was in his thousand-dollar suit so many months ago. His body was long, but muscular like a swimmer, and his perfect posture calmed the situation.

"Good morning," he said with a smile. "Are you guys ready?" he asked, as if we were about to step onto a roller coaster rather than into an operating room.

"I guess so," I responded, answering honestly. "More importantly, are you ready?" I asked in a poor attempt to inject levity to the situation and portray confidence to my wife.

"I am," he said, playing along with my game. He paused. "I know this is hard," he said looking at me first and then my wife, "but you're doing the right thing. I've got a great team in there and we are going to take great care of you." I appreciated his confidence.

"Okay, so now what we have to do is attach these green sensors to different parts of your face. The sensors will map your brain function through the surgery and help me navigate to the correct places in the brain." When he attached the green electrode to my face and scalp, oddly enough I felt like I was getting my face painted at a carnival. I looked pretty ridiculous and Kirstin and I took a selfie for posterity.

"All right," said Dr. Ross. "We are all done here. I've got to go to the operating room and set some things up. Once we are ready, I'll send Kimberly down to come get you. Kirstin, you can stay with him until we are ready."

"Thank you, doctor," Kirstin said, and he gave her a smile as he disappeared behind the curtain. We waited in relative silence, holding hands, with our foreheads touching at the point where the hairline meets the face. I was out of jokes and Kirstin was out of tears, so we just waited.

Right at 6:00 a.m., the advertised time of surgery, Kimberly knocked on the wall next to the curtain and asked, "Okay, Daniel. They are ready for you. Can I come in?" I responded in the affirmative.

"Mrs. Rufer, it's time for me to take Daniel back to the OR. Would you like me to show you to the waiting room?"

"No," she responded. "I can make it from here." She let go of my hands and hugged me hard around my upper back. "I love you," she said and kissed me softly on the lips. "Hot dog, ocean, golf."

"Hot dog, ocean, golf," I repeated to her and kissed her again. "I love you too. See you in a few hours." Kirstin kissed me one more time and slowly exited the room, leaving Kimberly and me alone. She passed me a tissue and I dabbed a tear from my eye.

"Are you ready?" she asked.

"Sure, where is the transport bed?"

"Oh, we don't do that for this type of surgery," she said picking up the slack from the dangling electrode cords. "We like to have patients walk into the OR. It gives them a greater orientation of where they are and outcomes are better."

"What if I pulled a runner right now? Has anyone ever done that?"

"No, you would be the first. You're not going to run, are you?" We exited the curtained room and the pre-op area. As we entered the main hallway, we turned away from the waiting area. I glanced inside to see if I could see Kirstin for a wave, but the glass window in the door only showed a small part of the room, and no one was occupying that space.

"I have to pee. I need to pee when I get nervous. Can I use the bathroom? What if I have to pee during surgery?" My head was suddenly spinning with questions and last-minute regret.

"There is a bathroom just up here on the left. You can use it, but wash your hands, and I'll be right outside." I entered the bathroom and locked the door behind me, trying to plot my various methods of escape. I looked at the air ducts. Too high. Then I remembered, Dr. Ross's statement that I was doing the right thing. I refocused and eked out three drops of urine before washing my hands and catching a glimpse of myself in the mirror. "Here, we go Daniel. No turning back now."

I exited the bathroom and Kimberly was waiting for me. "I washed my hands, I swear."

"I believe you. The OR is just a few doors up this way," she said as she extended her hand to the far end of the hallway. I followed her to the last door on the right and waited as she opened the door to what looked like a massive stainless-steel meat locker. I couldn't believe how huge the room was. If I had to guess, and I was only conscious in this room for about five minutes, I would say it was 40 feet wide by 40 feet long. I remember seeing three different operating tables towards the back of the room. Dr. Ross and four of his colleagues were huddled around a computer in the front left of the room. He appeared to be going over the game plan as a coach would with his players before a basketball game. The room was freezing. Not literally freezing, but certainly at a temperature well below 70. It was sweater weather in the OR, and I was wearing a paper-thin gown.

Kimberly politely led me to the far-left table and asked me to climb on board. Once I did, I was facing the grandeur of the operating room from the far-left corner. The anesthesiologist asked for my hand and I complied. "I'm going to start you on an IV to calm you down a bit and then we will administer the drugs that will put you to sleep." I wasn't listening to him, but I gave him my left arm. In addition to Dr. Ross, his four colleagues,

Kimberly, me, and this anesthesiologist, there were three additional nurses at the far end of the room. Even though I was the
one on the chopping block here, this was an impressive operation, pun intended. After another 30 seconds of taking it all in,
Kimberly squeezed my right hand and said, "You're going to do
great."

Channeling my father's quirky ability to tell a joke in an
uncomfortable situation, I said "It's not me I'm worried about."
Kimberly chuckled. I sat up and said, "Hey, Doc," in my best
teacher voice. I startled the anesthesiologist working on my left
side.

"Yes?" Dr. Ross said, looking up from his pregame huddle.
I motioned him over with my free arm.

When he stood before me I extended my right fist and
said, "Good luck out there today, doc." He forced an uncomfortable smile, reciprocated with a fist bump, and returned to the
huddle around the computer.

The anesthesiologist turned to me with a stern look and
said, "we really need to get started now." I nodded and lay back
to recline flatly on the operating table. "I'm going to count backwards from 10," he said "and I want you to do it with me." I
nodded.

"10, 9, 8,7." and the world went dark for the next 10
hours.

10 HOURS LATER...

If you've ever had surgery, you know that it is a disorienting experience. In most cases you go to sleep in one room, but you wake up in another. In this case, I fell asleep in the operating room expecting to wake up five hours later with a searing headache. Instead I woke up nearly 13 hours later with no headache, but with uncontrollable nausea and dizziness.

"Good evening, Daniel," a nurse said, though I couldn't focus my eyes enough to make out any features of this person. I was confused by her salutation because the surgery was only supposed to be five hours. "If you feel up for it, I will raise the top of your bed and you can see your family for a few minutes."

"Yes, please," I mumbled. The words were slurred and I was exhausted simply from moving my jaw. I tried to focus my eyes over the foot of my bed and out the window, which looked south. Everything was out of focus, blurry, and shaking back and forth. I only held that gaze for a few seconds, but I could tell that what the nurse was saying was true; evening was on its way. My surgery had lasted longer than five hours. I tried to close my eyes to preserve my energy, and it was then that I realized I could not close my right eye at all. This was an expected consequence of the surgery, but it is a strange feeling to be completely exhausted, want to bring your eyelid down, and be unable to do so. However, I noticed that with my left eye closed I was able to maintain single vision on the objects in the room. The vision out of my right eye was still shaky, but at least it was singular. I scanned the room from left to right, tilting my head in the process because this eye no longer had the ability to scan on its own. The lights in the recovery room were on, but dim. There was about two feet of room on both the left and right sides of my hospital bed and a couple feet at the foot of the bed. Over my feet, I could see a blue reclining chair, and beyond that a window, with the curtains open, that faced south. I could see the highway. The mix of white headlights and red taillights further confirmed that it was late in the day. I continued my scan to the right of the bed, where several instruments beeped and spat out information regarding my heart rate, blood pressure, and other things.

I heard a shuffle behind me and the nurse reappeared at my right side. "Your wife and family are here," she said, indicating with her eyes that they were on my left side. I tilted my head back to the left, keeping my left eye closed, to see my wife and parents. Kirstin had her hand firmly pressed on my left leg by the time I turned, but I felt nothing. "Hey, babe," my wife said. "Welcome back."

I labored to ask a question: "What time is it?" I sounded drunk, but only later would I come to understand that this was because only the left half of my face remained functional.

"It's about 8 o'clock. The surgery went longer than they thought, but everything went well. You look great," my wife strained to say. I was too tired to respond.

"You did great, Danny," chimed my mother. My father stood there with his arm on her shoulder.

"Okay, that's enough for now," interjected the nurse. "He needs to rest, but I'll come get you when the doctor comes for his visit."

"I love you," my wife said, squeezing my hand. She waited for me to squeeze back, but I couldn't feel anything on the left side of my body from my ear to my toe. When I saw her hand squeeze again, I responded by saying, "Hot dog, ocean, golf." She smiled and exited with my parents. I faded back into an exhausted sleep.

FOLLOW-UP

About two hours later, Dr. Ross arrived to check on me. The visit was a lot like the first time I saw him; he was wearing a well-cut suit and was trailed by a team of interns. "Hello Kirstin... Daniel," he said as he sidled up to the left side of the bed. The interns filled in behind my head and on my right side. Kirstin stood at the bottom left of my bed; she had apparently been sleeping on the blue recliner in the corner when Dr. Ross entered the room.

"How are you feeling?"

"Pretty terrible," I replied.

"I bet," he responded. "You had a very long and invasive surgery. Everything went well," he said, making sure to make eye contact with both me and my wife. "I'm confident that we got everything, but we are going to send you for an MRI tomorrow just to make sure." I was nonplussed by his excitement and I tried to focus on him using only my right eye. "I'm going to ask you to respond to a few tests and then we'll get out of here and let you rest." I would come to know these tests very well, as every doctor I would encounter over the next three weeks of hospitalization would ask me to perform these same tasks.

He extended his left index finger about two feet in front of my nose. "Try to follow my finger with both eyes." I obliged, but as soon as I opened my left eye the room began to spin and twist, like trying to focus a kaleidoscope. The sensation was disorienting and nauseating. I tried to follow his finger, but everything was a blur and in constant motion, up and down, left and right. I would later to come to understand that swelling in the brain caused my eyes to shake. The medical term for this is nystagmus. The degree of nystagmus I had in my left eye was like viewing the world after ten beers. It was probably only a six-beer effect in the right eye, but that eye viewed the world at a 30-degree pitch. Keeping both eyes open was an exercise in abstract art and only possible for the time it took to run these tests; any longer and I'd have to vomit.

Next, he asked me to smile. I obliged, and Dr. Ross stated something to his interns while pointing at the right side of my face. "Patient has partial paralysis of the right side." I couldn't tell at the time, but only my left cheek moved when I smiled. He asked me to raise my eyebrows. Same result. Movement on the left side only. He asked me to shut my eyes as tightly as I could. My left eyelid obliged, and my right remained open. This was the "buy-in" he was referring to when he proposed the surgery. It was scary, but because I was not looking into a mirror, I did not understand the extent to which my face was compromised at the time.

Far more terrifying was the complete lack of sensation that I was about to discover on the left side of my body. Dr. Ross took the tip of his retracted click-pen and began touching various parts of my body, starting with the bottom of my left foot. "Can you feel that?" I shook my head no. He did the same on the bottom of my right foot. "Can you feel that?" I nodded that I could.

He repeated the process with my left shin. "Can you feel that?" I shook my head no. He did the same on my right shin. "Can you feel that?" I nodded that I could. He repeated this process several more time until he had established that I couldn't feel anything on the left side of my body. The left side of my face pursed and a tear trickled out of my right eye.

"This is common, Daniel. You just went through a very serious surgery. You have a lot of swelling in your brain right now." He checked a drainage tube that was attached to the back of my skull. "You have a lot of healing to do, and decreased sensation in the areas affected by the surgery is common. You simply need to rest and the sensation will start to come back."

He was trying to be reassuring, but this was not like waiting for your hair to come in after a bad haircut. Half my face didn't work and 50 percent of my body was completely numb.

"I'll come to see you next week after the MRI and see how you are doing. Do you have any questions for me?" I had a million questions. I wanted to scream. I felt like I had made the biggest mistake of my life. I felt responsible for putting myself in this hospital bed. I was terrified, angry, and exhausted all at once.

I was able to eke out a feeble "no" while shaking my head and futilely trying to hold back tears. My wife rose to thank him for coming by, and the surgeon and his white-coat army left the room. Kirstin grabbed my left hand and pulled it to her face. We cried together until I fell back asleep.

EVERY HOUR

The intensive care unit is not a restful place. Even with a closed door, it is noisy and chaotic. Everything beeps or dings. Everyone who works there is in constant motion. And no matter what time of day it is, the ICU is alive with noise and movement.

Every hour on the hour, someone comes into your room and says the same thing: "Hello, my name is Audrey/Samantha/Betty and I'm here to take your vital signs." When you are drifting in and out of consciousness, the person who checks on you imprints no personality. You simply cannot remember what is happening. For the purposes of this book, I have assumed that all ICU nurses are 5'4" female brunettes with a slight New Jersey accent and dark-rimmed glasses. Every hour, on the hour, Audrey/Samantha/Betty would come into the room, introduce herself, check all the beeping and dinging machines, take my pulse, check the discharge tube hanging from the back of my head, give a polite smile, and leave. Wait one hour; rinse and repeat.

I only truly remember one check-in over the 30 or so hours I spent in the ICU. This nurse was a man. Let's call him John. That was probably not his name, but John is my father's name and I generally like people named John. It doesn't matter. I wasn't lucid and I would never be able to recognize anyone I met in the first four days after my surgery were I to pass them on the street. My visit with John was memorable only because he was there to remove a catheter that had been in place since the beginning of the surgery. Our visit was at some point in the middle of the day on Friday, June 26th, though I cannot recall the exact timing. I remember John explaining to me that he was there to remove a catheter and to see if I could urinate on my own. This was interesting news to hear given that I did not know a catheter was worming its way up my urethra and into my bladder. Until this moment I hadn't considered the functionality of my genitalia. In between fitful naps, I was certainly sad and aware of my newly horrible eyesight and the lack of feeling on the left side of my body, but it had not yet occurred to me that the numbness I was experiencing might extend all the way to my sexual organ as well. I tried to suppress my anxiety over the potential loss of my manhood and eloquently asked John: "Wait, so my dong doesn't work?"

John, trying to maintain professional integrity, explained, "We inserted a catheter during surgery. It's very common."

I replied that I couldn't feel half of my body. At that moment, John pulled the catheter from my urethra and asked me, "Can you feel that?"

I winced in pain and was simultaneously horrified and relieved. "Yes," I said, suppressing a few curse words.

"Your *dong* will be just fine," he said with a smile as he carried the used catheter and expelled urine bag toward the garbage. It was the first bit of physical pain I experienced post-surgery, but it was terrific.

NEURO STEP-DOWN

On Saturday, June 27th, I was moved to the neuro step-down unit on the fourth floor. It's sort of like hospital purgatory. It's the in-between floor that gets you from the noisy, miserable ICU experience to the less noisy, but still miserable neurology floor. In the ICU, only one person could be in the room at any time. In step-down, I remember passing most of the day with my parents and wife at my side. The room was bigger and could accommodate more chairs. In step-down, the nurse visits were less frequent (probably every other hour), but a bit more involved.

Here the nurses were less interested in keeping you alive--I was essentially out of the woods on that--and more interested in getting you moving. It was on this day, more than 48 hours after the commencement of the surgery, that I first attempted to get out of bed. I don't remember it at all, but it must have happened because I read about it in the "accomplishment journal" that my wife kept. Despite the exclamation point next to "Daniel walked," I don't think I got very far. I doubt I even left the room. Two days later, "peed standing up" is listed as an accomplishment, so I'm thinking Kirstin applied the term "walked" quite liberally.

The other big thing that I remember from the neuro step-down unit was my trip to the MRI machine. I couldn't get an MRI while I was in ICU because it was too dangerous, but now that I was in step-down, I was cleared for it. Because of my physical state, getting this postoperative MRI was a difficult task. It required two orderlies to move me into another bed and then place me on the MRI machine. Because of that, and because the hospital didn't want me waiting by the machine, it took nearly six hours for the procedure to get underway. They started getting me ready for the test around 6:00 p.m., but it didn't actually happen until a little past midnight.

I was still quite dizzy and nauseous when the orderlies came for me and rolled my bed to the elevator. I tried to keep my eyes closed as we rumbled down the hallways, but my right eye always remained open. I felt every divot in the floor, every door jamb, every speed up, every slow down, in the pit of my stomach. Luckily, I hadn't eaten for three days, so throwing up was not an option. Still, nausea without vomiting as a constant state of being is unpleasant.

After the orderlies left, a burly army sergeant-like woman came over to prep me for the test. "It'll be about five minutes. We are just finishing up with someone, and then you're up next." I didn't respond.

My wife said, "When we're ready to go in, can you tape his eyes shut? He gets very dizzy when they are open."

"We can do that." She turned to me.

Just then a different technician appeared directly over my face and asked, "You're not going to throw up, are you?" I tried to shrug. "You can't throw up once you're inside the machine." I nodded as if I had control over my nausea, but all this talk of vomit was making me feel more and more anxious.

A couple minutes later the technician returned with some gauze pads and surgical tape. "You're sure you want the tape?

"He wants the tape," my wife implored. I nodded slowly and closed my left eye.

With little regard for my fragile state, the female technician placed a gauze pad over my right eye and applied a long piece of tape vertically from my hairline to my cheek. She paused, looking down at me in a dejected way, like I was holding up traffic at a red light. "He can't close his right eye," Kirstin interjected, obviously irritated by this woman's callous manner. I pulled the gauze pad off my eye and softly pulled my top right eyelid down gently before reapplying the bandage with my right hand.

As if I had done something wrong, the technician asked, "Are we good?"

I nodded.

"Okay, Daniel. We are going to roll you over to the exam room and then my colleague is going to help me lift you onto the machine." I tried to steady my breathing to compensate for the fact that I felt as if I was on a pool raft in a churning ocean.

As we began rolling, Kirstin said, "I love you, honey. I'll be right outside." Then the door shut and the temperature dropped about fifteen degrees. We were now in the MRI room.

I heard footsteps approach from the right side of my body, but because only my left eye was open, I couldn't see what was happening in my (now permanent) blind spot. Hands grabbed the sheets from under my torso on both sides. A deep voice boomed: "Okay, on the count of three. One, two, three." Just then I felt myself being lifted and not-so-gently moved from the rolling gurney to a hard-plastic plank. This was the platform that would retract into the MRI tube for the test. My head was at the foot of the tube and the male voice explained that he would have to move me a little bit to position me correctly for the test. My right eye began to peel open, but I said nothing and tried to force it back closed. The two technicians worked quickly to stabilize my head with some kind of neck brace and to stabilize my body by strapping me to the machine. I could now see a little bit out of my right eye, and I asked if one of the technicians would try to fix it. The same forceful hand as before reached across my head, pressed my eyelid down, and tightened the tape on my forehead.

"Okay, now?" she asked, clearly frustrated by how difficult this scan was becoming.

"Yes," I replied, but my eyelid was already starting to peel open again.

The male technician spoke: "Okay, you have to be very still now. The more you move, the longer this will take. You have a button next to your right hand. If you need me to stop the scan, press the button. But try not to." I tried to slow my breathing. This was not going to be fun. "I'm going to slide you back into the machine now, okay?" I gave the thumbs up, even though I really wanted to scream, "Get this shit off of me."

The platform started to slide back into the machine. As my head passed into the tube, part of the gauze pad caught on the tube and peeled back over my eye, scraping the surface of my eye with its sterile but rough surface. It felt as my eye was being dragged over a sandy surface until the platform stopped moving. I winced in pain, and the male technician asked if I was okay. I responded that I was because I just wanted this over with, and I didn't imagine that he could or would better the situation. I gave a thumbs up and braced for the worst: thirty minutes of claustrophobic nausea with one eye searing from having just being scraped by a paper product, and now staring at the inside of the cream-colored MRI tube without the ability to alter my gaze, focus it, or even keep it steady.

The test lasted for what seemed like an eternity, though it probably was only 30 minutes long. I essentially held my breath every time the machine went on. The pulsing, buzzing, and clanking of the machine was so loud that I could feel it in my bones. Perhaps because of the swelling in my head, the buzzing of the machine made the nystagmus of my left eye even worse than before. So, for thirty minutes I lay there trying to think of a happy place, trying to picture the beach or find my inner penguin, but I was constantly pulled back to reality by the clanking of the machine and the uncontrollable fluttering of my eye. To make matters worse, about halfway through the scan I began hallucinating shapes and colors that rose and fell like waves in the ocean and moved from left to right. The hallucinations started as colored circles, like the ones you see when you rub your eyes while they are closed. A red or blue shape would shakily appear on the left side of my field of vision and flutter from left to right until it disappeared. Then another shape would appear and repeat the process. The shapes weren't anything particular, more like looking at moving clouds. After a while, though, the shapes gave way to what appeared to me as cream-colored worms that would start their migration across my field of vision every twenty seconds or so. And so, for the last ten minutes of this MRI I lay still, trying to convince myself the worms that appeared to be crawling out of the MRI machine just three inches from my face were not real.

When the test was over and the platform slid me out from inside the tube, the male technician said, "Hey, you should have told me the eye patch fell off. I woulda fixed it." I exhaled and waited to be bounced back to the neuro step-down unit. I was proud of myself for surviving this ordeal, but traumatized by the appearance of these hallucinations. I wondered if they were now part of my life.

DAYS THREE & FOUR

The third day of my "achievements notebook" simply reads "ate peaches and ice cream." This was significant because the peaches and ice cream I ate were the first solid foods I had eaten since the surgery. That is to say, I had not eaten any solid foods in the 72 hours since the start of brain surgery. Two days later, I would weigh myself at 160 pounds, 10 pounds lighter than when I entered the hospital on June 25th. Up until the third day after surgery and for a few days more, I was completely uninterested in food. I only ate because nurses and family members implored me to do so. Not only was I not hungry, but the room appeared on a thirty-degree tilt when viewed through my right eye and completely blurry and shaking when viewed through my left eye. Keeping both eyes open at the same time was not tolerable.

Days three and four of my recovery were not particularly remarkable. I spent those days in the regular neurological floor of the hospital, watching television and chatting with my family. I was awake for most of the daytime hours and asleep for most of the nighttime hours. The checks on my vitals were less and less frequent, and by day four I was existing in my hospital bed with no oxygen and no intravenous drugs. But I wasn't progressing in terms of strength, endurance, coordination, or sensation. The left side of my body from my ear all the way down to my toe was still completely numb. When the physical therapist came for their visits, I became painfully aware of just how deficient those 10 hours in the operating room had made me.

"Mr. Rufer, with your right eye only, please follow my index finger." The therapist would start in front of my face and drag their finger to my left, which I could follow, then to my right, which I could not. "Mr. Rufer, with your left eye only, please follow my index finger." The therapist would start in front of my face and drag it to my right, which I could follow, then to my left, which I could follow. However, when looking to the far left, my left eye would shake uncontrollably. This condition only dissipated to a functional level after a month of therapy. The inability of my right eye to "cross the midline" would never correct itself and would require surgery a year later. My eyes are/were far less affected in their vertical range.

"Mr. Rufer, with both your eyes open, please follow my index finger." I stopped responding to this question after the first two therapists asked me, because having both eyes open triggered a gag reflex. "Okay, Mr. Rufer, you can close both of your eyes now." I would then close my left eye and reach for an eye patch to cover the right one. "I'm going to use the side of this pen to press lightly on different parts of your body. When you feel something, I want you to say yes." The therapist would usually alternate touching the left side of my body in one place and the right side of my body in the corresponding place. They would usually start at the base of my foot and work their way up to my torso. Yes, no, yes, no, yes, no, yes, no. The pattern didn't change for the entire time I was on the sixth floor. I was told that increased numbness was common after a surgery such as mine. After all, numbness was the presenting symptom that led me down this path to begin with, so having it exacerbated by the surgery, while troubling, was not the most devastating disability I suffered. That title went to my loss of coordination.

I would then switch the patch to cover my left eye. "Mr. Rufer, I want you to extend the pointer finger on your right hand like I'm doing and tap my finger as I move it around in the air." With my right hand extended, I could tap the therapist's finger with my own the requisite eight times as it revolved around my field of vision. "Okay, Mr. Rufer, now I want you to extend the pointer finger on your left hand like I'm doing and tap my finger as I move it around in the air." Miss, miss, miss, miss, miss,

60

miss, miss, miss. It wasn't just missing the target that was upsetting. It was the *way* I missed that was so devastating. On top of having no sensation in my left hand whatsoever, I also couldn't hold it steady for even a second. Imagine extending your arm to point at something with your index finger, only to find that your entire arm was shaking like a flag in a stiff breeze. My left arm shook when it was extended. It shook when I was moving it vertically. It shook when I was moving it horizontally. The only time it didn't shake was when it was resting at my side. I had acquired a Parkinson's-like shake to my left arm overnight. When the therapist asked me to touch my finger to my nose with my right hand, I did it easily. When, he asked me to do it with my left hand, I missed by two feet. The gravity of my situation was starting to set in.

THE MOVE TO REHAB

Around noon on day five, I moved to a different part of the hospital: the rehabilitation center. It was both a relief and a hardship to complete the move. On the rehab floor I would be given more autonomy. It would be quieter. And I could finally get down to the business of recuperation. When I was wheeled into room 1625, I was greeted with a loud hello from my new roommate, Marco, who was recovering from spinal fusion surgery. Marco was a small 80-year-old man of Italian descent who was never at a loss for words.

"You're way too young to be in here, kid!"

I laughed. "I had brain surgery last Thursday. I'll be in here for four or five days."

"Yeah, that's what they told me," he said dejectedly.

"How long have you been here?"

"Two weeks."

"Huh." I had no response to that.

Marco occupied the bed on the far side of the room, near the window. I would occupy the bed closest to the hallway and the bathroom. He was more able than I was at the outset, plus he had been there longer, so he had dibs on the view. As I tried to settle my eyes in his general direction I noticed that Marco wasn't wearing a blue shirt, but a blue jersey of the hated New England Patriots. "I have to give you fair warning, Marco." He twisted slightly in his wheelchair to hear me better. "I don't take kindly to Patriots fans."

He laughed a little and then winced in pain. "It hurts to laugh sometimes. I'm actually a Giants fan, but Teddy Bruschi is my nephew."

"Oh," I said reluctantly. "He's probably the only Patriot I even remotely like. He was a tough player. He's good on NFL Live. Do we get ESPN up here?"

"I watch it every day at 4:00 p.m."

"Great. At least we have that in common." As soon as I finished my sentence, his daughter entered the room behind me, carrying what looked like a delicious sandwich.

"Ciao, Giulia, this is...?" Marco trailed off, making his statement a question.

"Daniel."

"Hello, I am Giulia. I am Marco's daughter," she said with a thick Italian accent.

I managed to say "Nice to meet you" before she turned away from me and began lecturing her father in Italian. As the conversation turned more heated, she pulled the curtain that divided the room. I'm not sure what they were talking about, but if I had to guess, I'd bet she was angry with him for getting out of bed without help. In the four days I had Marco as a roommate before he transferred to another room under the cover of darkness because I "snore like a rhinoceros," I would observe his relationship with his daughter as more mother-son than father-daughter.

A few minutes after the orderly settled me into bed, my parents arrived with some matzo ball soup from a nearby deli. I wasn't hungry, but I appreciated the sentiment. "Looks like you've got a roommate," my mother said as she bent over to kiss me on the cheek and set the soup down on my tray.

"Yeah, his name is Marco. And he's a Patriots fan." Marco responded by saying *ciao*. My father jokingly called for the nurse to transfer this "traitor" from the hospital. Thankfully, no one heard his plea. "Easy, dad. I just got here. Plus, he had spinal fusion surgery just like you."

"Oh, really?" My father's interest was piqued, and he knocked on the wall next to the curtain before peering over to Marco's area. "Who was your surgeon?" And they were off and running in a conversation only two old men could have.

My father reemerged a couple minutes later and took a seat at the edge of bed. "Nice guy. I always liked Teddy Bruschi." A few more minutes passed and I continued not to eat the soup that was bought for me. By then, the hospital-provided lunch had arrived and I managed to eat two saltines and drink half a cup of apple juice over the course of the next 30 minutes. Giulia and Marco were arguing again, as would become the pattern. Twenty minutes of peaceful conversation followed by five minutes of yelling and usually a few exasperated sighs from Giulia and a weak smack of the bedside tray from Marco. I had no idea what they were talking about, but it was always entertaining.

Around 1:00 p.m., Kirstin arrived from work, carrying a salad in one hand and her purse in the other. "This room is much easier to find than the other," she said, and gave me a soft kiss on the cheek. "How's it going?" she asked as she placed her bag on my bed and the salad on my tray before turning to hug each of my parents.

I responded that it was good to be on a different floor and that I liked my new roommate.

"Oh, you have a roommate?" she said, and peeked around the curtain. "I'm Kirstin, Dan's wife."

Marco said hello and Giulia said *ciao*. Then the two continued their conversation, rapidly firing off words in Italian at varying volumes and emphasis. Kirstin tried to ignore their conversation to ask me about the new bed. Did I know what else was on this floor? Had I seen anyone yet?

My answers were all short and devoid of information. Right before she settled onto the corner of my bed, she said, "Excuse me," and walked out into the hallway. We could hear her sobbing and a nurse trying to console her.

My father asked quietly, "What was that about?"

"Our honeymoon. We would have been in Rome today if it weren't for the surgery." My dad looked confused, but my mother understood exactly what I meant and went into the hallway to console Kirstin. After five days of trying to adjust to hospital visits being normal, we were confronted immediately, through no fault of our own, with exactly what our life was not. We were not on our honeymoon. We were not dreaming of a future with a beautiful home, three children, and 2.5 cars. We were in a hospital room trying to put on a good face about the fact that our entire future had been altered by one tiny vascular anomaly, and trying somehow and some way to make believe that things were going to be okay. At that moment, the differences between what was and what could have been were crystal clear and excruciatingly saddening.

DAY ONE

The 15 days I spent in rehab were the most physically and mentally grueling days of my life. A typical day in rehab consisted of two 30-minute PT sessions, two 30-minute OT sessions, and one 30-minute speech session. To readers, two and a half hours of mild physical activity might not seem like a lot, but I can attest to the fact that, coming off of a 10-hour brain surgery, it was completely exhausting.

As stated in the previous chapter, I arrived on a Tuesday around noon, so my first day in rehab consisted only of the afternoon sessions. I remember being excited by the challenge of rehab. When I was settled on the sixth floor, I was evaluated for inpatient rehab and it was recommended that I complete between two and three weeks of inpatient therapy before I could return home. Having played sports my entire life, including collegiate baseball, I was ready to prove any doubters wrong. In sports, you tackle whatever barriers exist in front of you. In college, it took me two years to elevate myself from walk-on outfielder with a decent arm who never played on a lousy team to the number two starting pitcher on a decent (but not great) team. I was used to the doubt; I enjoyed the challenge. I liked to push my body, be it on the mound or the gym. I had lost twenty pounds in the build-up to my wedding, sported a 31-inch waist, and kept my weight at pre-college levels all the way up until the surgery. I was ready for this challenge and I was ready to prove the experts wrong.

Then reality set in. In my first PT session, I was tasked with getting up from a seated position. It wasn't easy and was compounded by the fact that I still couldn't feel anything in my left leg or hand. A primary concern of mine (and the therapists) was that I would sit on my hand or bang it into something without noticing because I couldn't feel it or sense its general location in space. (The term for this ability, which I would later learn, is proprioception.) I thought I was actually doing quite well in this activity, but Chandra, the therapist, told me I was leaning heavily to my right side both on the way up and the way down. To help me understand what I could not feel or perceive, she went to get a standing mirror and placed it three feet in front of me. As soon as I looked up, I lost it. I started sobbing. These were not modest, I'm-trying-not-to-cry tears. These were big, chest-heaving sobs of despair. What Chandra didn't know--couldn't have known, really--was that I hadn't seen myself in the mirror since the surgery.

I remember it vividly. I was wearing grey shorts and a bright green tank top. I was pale and skinnier than I had been since grade school. My arms were littered with bruises from different IVs and I was hunched over and listing 20 degrees to the right. I couldn't perceive the tilt of my head even as I looked at myself. My face was ashen and my mouth drooped heavily on the right side. Since I was wearing an eye patch over my left eye and my right eye was stuck motionless and pointed inward over my nose, my head was rotated to the right to compensate for my new and altered line of sight. In short, I didn't recognize myself, and it was devastating. I looked away from the mirror and crumpled on the bench where we were working. I explained to Chandra that I hadn't seen myself in the mirror since before the surgery and cried in her lap for at least ten minutes. That was the beginning (and end) of my first day of therapy. Chandra cancelled the rest of my session for the day and I was wheeled back to my room, where I fell asleep until the hospital dinner arrived. That was what I refer to as Day One.

DAY TWO

Thursday, July 1st began with a manicure. After a virtually untouched breakfast, I was brought via wheelchair to the rehab center.

"Red, green or blue?" Chandra asked, holding three different types of nail polish in her left hand.

"Um, none. I'm not really good at fashion advice."

"Not for me, Daniel. This is for you." I shook my head in disbelief. "We are going to paint the nails on your left hand so you can see them better--so you can get a better sense of where your hand is spatially."

"Oh, that makes sense. I had a catcher in college that used to do that. It made it easier to see the signals. He wore white."

"We don't have white," she said, holding up the three options.

"Well, I think I'm too pale for red, and that blue is too dark, so let's go with the green. Let's go with green. It will irritate my roommate Marco, who is a stupid Patriots fan." I said the last part loudly for Marco's benefit, but he was off in some other part of the room using one of the treadmills. I would needle him about the green nail polish later in the day, but without much satisfaction.

While Chandra was painting my nails she said, "I'm sorry about yesterday. I didn't... I didn't know that you hadn't--"

"It's okay. This is just way harder than I thought. I'd been avoiding mirrors for the past few days. It's time to start moving forward."

"Well that's the right attitude," she said, finishing my pinky finger. "Wave that--" meaning my hand--"around for a few minutes while I get set up over there, and I'll be right back."

While I waved my newly lime green nails in a completely uncoordinated circle, I took stock of the room that would become my gymnasium for the next two weeks. It was a large open space that ran the complete width of the building, approximately 50 feet. The inpatient rehab room was shaped like the letter "u," with the entrance coming at the top of the middle part of the letter and opening up to workstations to the left and the right. Because the hospital was situated in the far East Side of Manhattan and because we were on a high floor of that building, there was a tremendous (sometimes blinding) amount of light in the room. The longest edge of the room faced east and thus was very bright in the morning hours. But given the drudgery of what each of us was trying to accomplish, it was nice to have a decent view to counteract the monotony and frustration.

Situated around the room were four eight-foot-by-eight-foot mechanical mats, upon which therapists could stretch patients and/or guide them in abdominal planks, push-ups, sit-ups, or basically any other frustrating callisthenic exercise. The mechanical aspect of these mats is quite ingenious, because the therapist can support the patient in a floor exercise without actually having to get on the floor. The mats were usually suspended 18 inches above the ground, but depending upon the height of the patient or the activity in question, they could be raised or lowered by up to a foot. Continuing to scan the room, I found a treadmill, an exercise bike, a shoulder bike, racks and racks of therapy balls, and one set of parallel bars, which would become the bane of my existence in a few days.

Most of the patients on this floor were, like Marco, older men. Many of them had experienced a stroke, a fall, or a back injury that had left them immobile enough that they, like me, had to learn how to walk again. I would estimate that at this time there were 20 patients in rehab. We were a motley crew. Only four of the patients were women, and I'd guess that there were only two other people who, like me, were under 40. One was a woman in her early thirties who had just had both hips replaced to offset a degenerative disease. The other was a man, who, like me, had had brain surgery to remove a tumor. His surgery was in a less vulnerable part of the brain and he was already walking without a cane by the time I arrived on the rehab floor. Our time in rehab only overlapped for a few days, but seeing someone at the other end of recovery gave me hope.

"Okay, Dan." Chandra had returned. "We're going to start with ten squats like we did yesterday, but this time without the mirror." I nodded and received help from one of the assistants to walk from the wheelchair to the mat. He was a hulking man with a 6'3 frame, probably weighing over 250 pounds. As I stood up, he grabbed my left arm just above the elbow and pulled upward to help me stagger the ten or so steps to the mechanical exercise mat. Upon my arrival at the mat, I tried to rise from the seated position, but instead pushed myself diagonally to the left. Chandra caught me and helped me back down to the mat before I could fall.

"Okay, Dan. I appreciate your enthusiasm, but you're going to have to let me get in position before we start any exercise. We don't want you falling." The notion that I could fall had not really occurred to me, even though the nurses always talk about "not falling." The rehab floor had a "no falls since" chart across from the nurses' station. The number of days was something like 11. I had no way of knowing whether or not that number was good or bad, but Chandra was right, I needed to slow down. The ten steps from the wheelchair to the mechanical mat had made me tired, and I asked for a cup of water. After I hydrated, caught my breath, and Chandra was in position, I rose slowly for the ten squats. Next, we did a toe tapping exercise and a few upper body stretches. Before I knew it, the thirty-minute session was over and I was introduced to Lauren, who would be my occupational therapist while in the hospital.

Lauren often joked that I was her "left hand man," a cringeworthy play on the colloquialism right-hand man. I protested the label as misleading, since a left-hand man would likely be untrustworthy. My pleas for a more apt nickname notwithstanding, Lauren tried to force me to do everything with my left hand, from opening doors to cutting food to playing checkers. Everything I was challenged to do with my left hand was difficult. When we started, the fine motor skills that you need to type or use a remote were gone (they still are), but at the beginning I had no gross motor skills either. My left hand shook so much that tapping an area the size of a deck of cards was nearly impossible. (Now I'm pretty good at pushing elevator buttons, but drinking a glass of water with my left hand is still not possible.)

The third therapy stop for the morning was to see the speech therapist, Nancy. As you can imagine, Nancy and I practiced talking. My pronunciation has certainly gotten better over the past two years, but it wasn't all that terrible even five days after the surgery. The words that give me trouble now are the words they gave me trouble then. Words that start with the letter "f" are the most difficult to pronounce. To form the correct sound for the letter "f," one needs to tuck the lower lip under your top teeth. Because I only have control over half of my face, only half of my lower lip is able to create that sound correctly. For that reason, the "f" sound I now make is slightly slurred and delayed in its delivery. To this day, I try not to assign math problems in the forties or fifties because it creates problem for me when it comes time to read from the answer key in class. In a typical session, Nancy would assign me a bank of words to practice pronouncing. She would also challenge me to hold my breath or speak at a loud volume. Speech therapy was certainly the least taxing of all my normal 30-minute sessions, but at this point, five days out from surgery, even practicing pronunciation wiped me out. On the first day, I was returned to my room around 10:30 a.m. Once back in bed, I immediately fell asleep and stayed so until I was awoken at 1:00 p.m. for the afternoon sessions.

HOWARD J

The first non-familial guest to visit me in the hospital was my father's best friend, certified nutjob, and fellow Jets fan Howard J. My father, Howard, Howard's son, and I have shared season tickets to the New York Jets for over 20 years. The four of us have attended nearly every Jets home game since the 1995 season. I am absolutely certain of the start date because Howard is a dead ringer for the Jets' head coach during that dismal season (Rich Kotite) and the fans in our section always used to give him grief about it. For those without a mental image of Rich Kotite, picture Larry David with a retired Florida tan and a healthy paunch belly.

"What's up, young man?" boomed Howard as he entered the hospital room. It took a moment for the smell of greasy diner food to follow him into the room. He placed a brown paper bag filled with assorted artery-clogging food items from a local Jewish deli on the adjustable tray. "I like the pirate thing you've got going on. Is it hard to have sex with one eye?" Howard is the kind of guy that can get away with saying just about anything, no matter how racy, and making it seem hilarious.

After a long pause, I replied, "I have no response to that. Thanks for coming."

"Of course. Your dad told me what happened and I would have come sooner, but he told me to wait a few days. How long do they think you'll be in here?"

"Two weeks, but I'm hoping for less. Would you mind moving this tray over near the sink? It's making me nauseous."

"Okay, but you gotta eat, Daniel. You're skin and bones. I've got the pastrami, corned beef, fries, knish. I know you like a knish." I felt a swell in the back of my throat.

"Maybe later. It's been a long day and I haven't been eating much."

"I can see that." Earlier in the day, a nurse checked the scale on my bed. I was down to 160 pounds, ten pounds lighter than I was five days ago. "Where's Kirstin?"

"She's at work, but she should be here soon." Kirstin had stopped sleeping at the hospital once I was moved to the rehab center. For these two weeks on the 16th floor, Kirstin slept at home, but visited every day from 6:00-9:00, and longer on Sundays. I can't imagine what it must have been like for her: visiting her crippled husband every evening and going home to an empty apartment. It was around this time that our dog started sleeping in our bed, a situation that has continued to this day.

"So, have you guys had any conjugal visits since the surgery?"

"First of all, this isn't a prison," I said, trying not to laugh. "And second of all, I have a roommate." Howard peeked behind the curtain. Marco must have been sleeping, because Howard then whispered in a stern tone, "A fucking Pats fan. No, no, no. This cannot stand. First brain surgery and then they stick you with a guy from Boston. This is fucked up. I'm going to talk to the head nurse." And he got up to exit the room. I truly think he was going to ask to get me transferred, because that's the kind of thing Howard would do, but just then my wife walked into the room.

"Howard, glad you could make it." They exchanged a hug and Kirstin kissed me on the cheek. She was still warm from the overbearing heat outside.

"They've got him shacked up with a Patriots fan. He can't heal in an environment like this. I'm going to go the nurses' station and get this sorted out."

Before he could leave, my wife interjected that it would be okay, that I was happy in this room and not to disturb the nurses with this. Kirstin has a way of defusing boisterous people, usually men, and putting them in their place. Howard retreated to a chair at the end of the bed, defeated but respectful of my wife's wishes.

That lasted about ten seconds.

"So, Daniel tells me that you haven't bumped uglies since the surgery."

Kirstin shot him a death stare and a smile and said, "Why don't we go down the hall for a while and let Marco rest?" Kirstin lowered the bed, locked the wheelchair, and Howard grabbed me under the arm to help me out of bed. The three of us traveled down the hall to the visitors' lounge, where an expansive view of downtown Manhattan lay before us. Howard emptied the contents of the food bag onto a table. "You've got to eat something, young man. I can't finish this myself," he said, chomping into a massive pastrami sandwich.

"He's right, Danny. You haven't eaten anything in five days. Just try a little." Kirstin undid one of the pastrami sandwiches and laid out a bite-size portion of pastrami for me to try. I acquiesced to the peer pressure and placed a small piece of pastrami onto my tongue.

To my surprise, it was amazing. The salty-soft meat awoke something in my body. I wasn't hungry per se, but addicted. It was like the first time I had a Dorito, but times ten. "Pass the mustard, please." I pulled the aluminum tin closer to me and began tearing away ever-larger pieces of pastrami, dipping them in mustard before shoveling them into my mouth. Then I tried a French fry and some corned beef. Rediscovering eating was so freeing… and probably disgusting to watch.

After a couple minutes of watching me devour cured meat and fried potatoes, Kirstin pulled the plate away from me. "That's enough for now." I slumped sadly. I hadn't felt alive like that in days. The food, albeit salty and cholesterol-packed, gave me energy and vigor.

And that was the day that I went from losing weight at an incredible rate to gaining it.

SHOWER TIME

Thursday, July 2nd began with a 5:00 a.m. wake-up call for a shower. Every patient had to shower every day. But every patient on this floor needed help showering. So, every patient had to sign up for a shower time with the nurses' station before dinner. Showers were either offered after 8:00 p.m. or before 7:00 a.m. Because I was new, I was one of the last to pick, and so I was awakened from fitful sleep at 5:00 a.m. by a male nurse. Let's call him Jim.

The halogen lights slammed on for my side of the room only (Marco was a night showerer). " Good morning, Mr. Rufer," Jim said, looking down at my chart. "Are you ready to take a shower?"

"No," I grunted.

Unamused, Jim replied, "Okay, I can come back after I have helped all the other patients."

"No, no, no. Wait. I'm ready," I said as I pushed myself up into a sitting position.

Showering is perhaps the most dangerous thing a patient can do while in a hospital. The risk of falling when your balance and strength are compromised is only exacerbated by wet and slippery surfaces. On day seven, I wasn't yet doing much of anything on my own, so it took Jim on one side and another nurse on the other side to help me out of bed and into the bathroom/shower. Like a shower one might use on a boat, the bathroom that I shared with Marco had a drain in the center of the floor. The toilet was directly across from the entrance and the larger shower area was off to the right, separated by a curtain that was pulled all the way back. In the middle of the shower area was a toilet-seat-high-chair that was used by patients for whom the regular toilet was too low to the ground. There was no plumbing attached to this device and I quickly realized that it was going to be my "shower chair" for today. Once I was placed into the chair, Jim gave me a moment to catch my breath and the helper nurse left. "When you are ready I want you to stand up by holding the bars on both sides." I took a deep breath and followed his instructions. Once in a standing position, my left leg began to rock, and I was forced to sit back down. I didn't yet have the strength to stand for any measurable period of time. "You okay?" Jim asked. I nodded and tried again. I rose out of my seat, rocking back and forth until I was standing still and tall. It didn't last long, but it was enough time for Jim to untie my robe and pull down my underpants. Once I sat down, still clenching to the support bars with all my strength, he pulled the gown forward and off each arm. Next, he lifted each leg and removed each of my hospital-issued booties until I was completely naked, sitting on a railing-protected commode with no bottom. Jim then started the water on the shower handle. After he let the water run for a few seconds and he felt it himself, he splashed a little on my right leg and asked if the temperature was okay.

"A little warmer, please," I replied. He obliged and put the shower handle in my right hand and a washcloth and a bar of soap in my left hand.

"I'm going to leave you to it, but if you drop anything, pull on this cord here," he said, gesturing to the red emergency cord next to the temperature dial. "Don't reach for it. You WILL fall," he said emphatically. He was right. I nearly fell out my wheelchair the day prior reaching for my shoelace. I nodded that I understood and Jim left the room, dubious of my agreement.

After he left, I was both excited and scared. This was my first "real" shower in seven days. Every previous day I had been given a sponge bath, which is both ineffectual and freezing because the temperature in the hospital seems to always hover in the mid-60's. I raised the shower head to the side of my face and let it trickle down my back. The warm water felt incredible. Next, I let it pour over my chest and over my genitals. Then I raised my wobbly left arm to the ceiling and sprayed water into my left armpit. It was better than any outdoor shower might feel after a day at the beach. Next, I transferred the shower head to my left hand carefully and gripped it tight as I raised my right arm toward the ceiling for some underarm cleaning, but before the water reached my body, the showerhead slipped out of my left hand and slammed back into the wall to which it was attached. Having no sensation in my left hand meant that I often couldn't tell how hard I was holding things. My wife and I put a temporary moratorium on holding hands because I often crushed hers in mine without knowing it. But the problem worked both ways, and even though I thought I was gripping the showerhead tightly, I was not. After it clanged on the tile wall, it swung slightly closer to me. After a couple more swings, I was able to reach forward to snag the showerhead with my right hand. Unfortunately, when I did so both washcloth and soap fell to the floor. Happy that I had the showerhead, but realizing that I had used up my good fortune, I pulled the emergency cord. A minute or so later, Jim came back into the bathroom and saw the soap on the floor.

"Okay," he said. He picked up the soap and cloth and began scrubbing my chest and back with no particular gentleness. He then got under my arms and each of my legs. Then he said, "You see that bar on this wall?" He was referring to the support bar on the same wall as the showerhead. I nodded that I did. "You're going to stand up and grab that bar and stand for thirty seconds while I clean your backside." I was both embarrassed at the prospect of this stranger touching my private parts and nervous that I couldn't stand for that long. I think he could see the trepidation in my eyes when he said, "Don't worry, I'm not going to let you fall."

On three, two, one, I pushed off the support bars and stood before taking two shuffle-steps toward the wall in front of me. I grabbed the bar and held on for dear life, as if hurricane winds might come blowing in at any second. With much more gentleness, he scrubbed the outside of my thighs before lightly swabbing at my penis and testicles. It was probably not enough to clean that area after seven days, but I appreciated his discretion. He took one quick wipe of my backside before helping me back to the commode/shower chair. I sat there, exhausted but feeling clean for the first time in seven days, as Jim poured water on my hair and over the open wound at the back of my skull. "We need to clean this gently," he said, massaging my scalp. "You know this is going to get easier, right? This is not forever."

I shrugged, feeling defeated, as he turned off the water and began to pat me dry. "How long have you been here, a week? You're young," he said. "You'll get over this." I appreciated his positive outlook, but it was hard to feel positive about the future when your testicles only got cleaned once a week and by a stranger. He was correct though; things would get better. Jim helped me into some underwear, shorts, socks, and a shirt before getting me back in bed. The whole ordeal only took twenty minutes, but I was exhausted, and as soon as I got back in bed I fell asleep until the breakfast cart arrived.

"Hang in there, Mr. Rufer," he said as he left the room.

DAY 3: EVERY DAY IS THE SAME... SOMETIMES

Day 3 on the rehab floor established the beginning of what would become my routine for the next fourteen days. Shower at 5:00 a.m., return to bed for a nap, breakfast at 7:00 a.m., nap until first PT session, participate in physical therapy, participate in occupational therapy, return to room for nap, lunch at 12:30, nap until second PT session, participate in physical therapy, participate in occupational therapy, participate in speech therapy, return to room for afternoon nap, eat dinner at 7:00 p.m., visit with wife and/or friends and/or watch *Alaskan Bush People* on the Discovery Channel, fall asleep at (or before) 10:00 p.m. Wake up and do it again the next day.

Most PT sessions were focused on my lower body and my balance. While there was some practice walking, most of the therapy sessions were spent doing squats, toe taps, and leg raises. Most OT sessions were focused on my upper body deficiencies. Lauren would have me sort a deck of playing cards or transfer paper clips from one bowl to another. The *Rocky IV* montage it was not. That said, the therapists and other assistants were very kind, sometimes funny, always positive, and often cognizant of the monotony. About a week into my stay, while I was at one end of the therapy room sorting coins, a woman of about 60 emerged from the doorway with a long neon-colored rope.

"Here you go," she said dispassionately, handing it off to one of the therapists, who thanked the woman and examined the length of the rope. A few moments later, the therapist rose from her chair, walked over to an old fragile man in a wheelchair, and put the rope on his lap. She whispered something in his ear that I couldn't quite hear from my distance and wheeled him back into the center of the room. Once the wheels were locked, she walked around the front of his chair and summoned two orderlies for help. She then crouched down in front his chair and began to unfurl the brightly colored rope until all that was left in the old man's lap was a black handle, which he gripped very tightly. She gave instructions to both the patient and the orderly that I couldn't hear and stepped about ten feet away. She looked back toward the man still seated in his chair and with a slight pause said, "Okay," and began to pull strongly on the rope. The old man held on with all his might and within a few seconds had stood out of his chair with a smile ear-to-ear and the kind of groan that an excited baby might make.

This man, in his early 80s, had suffered a massive stroke that left his extremities severely compromised and, to the best of my knowledge, he no longer had the ability to speak. I hadn't quite noticed him before this moment except to note that he was probably in the worst shape of any of us on the rehab floor. It turns out that for all of his adult life, including the summer before this stroke, this skinny, hunched-over, wrinkled man had been quite the expert water-skier. His therapist, sensing a bit of a plateau with respect to his recovery, asked his wife about her husband's interests. When she replied that he was an avid water-skier, the therapist came up with the half-baked idea of recreating that feeling for him. With much doubt, the younger, but not young, wife retrieved a water-ski rope from their country home and brought it to the hospital. The indifference with which she dropped off the rope was replaced with exuberance and tears of joy as she hugged her husband on equal footing for the first time in over a month.

DAY 4: LUNCH WITH RYAN AND ERIC

    It's not as if I hadn't had any visitors thus far. My parents had been to see me multiple times. My in-laws were there in the immediate aftermath of the surgery. Howard came by on Wednesday to jumpstart my appetite but, to my recollection, I had successfully kept my friends at bay thus far. When Ryan and Eric came to visit, it represented a different type of interaction. All the previous visitors knew what I was going through. They were in the know from at least the time that surgery became a reality. Ryan and Eric, the first baseman and left fielder on my summer softball team, did not know what I was going through. Our season was about a month old and I hadn't played in any games, but I just shrugged it off (to others) as a lower-back injury and kept the neurological truth to myself. Once I was a couple days out from surgery and moved to the rehabilitation floor, I let Dave (my friend from the bar in the first chapter, and our center fielder) notify the team that I had in fact undergone brain surgery and would be recovering in the hospital for another couple of weeks. I'm not sure how Dave relayed that information, but texts and emails started pouring in from concerned teammates. I didn't respond to many at this point because a) I didn't want to and b) I couldn't focus my eyes on screens very well. On day 4 of rehabilitation (day 7 post-surgery), my eyesight was still quite poor. Not only did my eyes not work together, but my left eye still shook when I tried to focus it. This phenomenon made it quite nauseating to try to do anything with my left eye, so most of the time in the hospital I patched my left eye and used my right eye. My right eye didn't shake, but it also didn't move much. The cranial nerve that controlled aural movement (movement toward the ear or to the right) of my right eye had been severed in the surgery. The right eye could successfully hold a gaze, but it was functioning at a much lower level. I went into surgery will two eyes working together, but came out with two eyes that didn't work together, one of which shook uncontrollably and the other of which didn't move, was pointed inward, down, and only measured at 20/80 vision. Thankfully, my left eye would eventually recover to 20/20 status and would be (mostly) nystagmus-free, but at this time, my right eye was the best that I had. It pointed inward, forced me to turn my head 30 or so degrees to the right and 20 or so degrees to my right shoulder to look at someone or something head on. Bottom line: in the early days, my vision was horrible, and 21st-century communication was not high on my list of things to do.

When Eric and Ryan entered the hospital room, I was asleep from a morning of toe tapping and card-sorting. Ryan shook the bottom of my left leg and, though I didn't feel it, the rocking of the bed woke me from my slumber. By his voice, I could tell who was there, but I still needed a few seconds to refocus my right eye with a saline drop so that I could see them.

"Hey guys, thanks for coming. Sorry that I was asleep, but pretty much everything makes me tired."

"Don't worry about it, Dan. We're just glad you're okay," Ryan said in the calm tone of a caring father, which he was. Ryan had two children under the age of three and lived in Connecticut, but still found time to stop by the hospital on his first week of summer vacation. "I brought you some chicken soup," Ryan said, checking off all the boxes for the stereotypical friend-in-hospital visit. Never mind that I couldn't really taste anything, because the surgery had temporarily damaged some of the sensory nerves that control smell and taste. Most food nauseated me and if I was going to eat something, it had to be salty to be appetizing.

"Thanks, Ryan. Can you put it over there?" I said, pointing

to the roll-up tray that was a couple feet from my bed.

Eric, who had been standing behind Ryan for the exchange of pleasantries, walked around to the foot of my bed and with a made-for-TV smile said, "This room's not bad." He peered past the curtain that divided my side from Marco's. "And the view's pretty great." Eric was clearly forcing some small talk to avoid confronting his wounded softball buddy. "Why don't you just move over here?" Eric said, pulling back the curtain. It was then that I noticed that Marco had left me. Initially, I was happy for him, but that faded when I found out he moved to avoid my snoring.

"Huh," I said. "There was someone there this morning."

"Well, there's no one there now. Want me to ask if you can move over to the other side?"

"Yeah, that would be great, Eric. The nurses' station is out to the--"

"I got it. I saw it on the way in." Eric responded while he exited the room, taking the opportunity to leave the uncomfortable situation.

Upon Eric's return, the two of them lifted me out of bed and pushed me in a wheelchair to the guest visiting room, where they ate lunch and I tried not to vomit at the sight of food. They told me about the team and how the season wasn't the same without me. I appreciated the sentiment and told them that I'd be back for the playoffs, though I'm sure they knew that was not going to happen. Like Ryan, Eric was a new father, but his child was essentially a newborn. Over lunch, he told me about his son's vestigial tail and the tests that were being run. I didn't know much of anything related to his son's condition, but it sounded scary, and Eric tried to confidently say that everything was alright. (Everything would be fine with regard to his son). Ryan and Eric clearly had a lot going on in their lives, and it meant a lot to me that they stopped by for a visit. By the time they had finished their sandwiches and wheeled me back into the room, the window bay had been prepared for me. My softball buddies picked me up and dropped me in my new bed.

I thanked them for coming. Ryan offered the soup to me one more time, but I waved him off. I fell back to sleep by the time they made it to the elevator.

DAY 5: INDEPENDENCE DAY AND A HOT DOG

In 2015, Independence Day fell on a Saturday. Given that Sundays were always a day off at this rehab facility, it was a little wonky that I would get a two-day reprieve from treatment, but I had plenty of "homework" to do. At this time, most of my homework pertained to eye and face movement because (much to my frustration) it wasn't safe for me to even stand unsupervised.

The eye exercises were tedious, but important. I could already feel my vision improving, albeit slowly. The basic exercises at this time were following a finger or object with one eye. It didn't really matter what it was or where it moved as long as I concentrated intently on the moving object. On the rehab floor, it was usually a brightly-colored tongue depressor, but left to my own devices I would usually just stick my thumb out in front of my nose and move it from left to right, then up and down at varying degrees. I'd have Siri set a 60-second timer for the left eye, then pause for a moment and switch the eyepatch over and do it with the right eye. 60 seconds at a time until fatigue or boredom won out.

As for arm exercises, I was supposed to move and stack three plastic cups on my roll-up tray. Honestly, I think I only did this once or twice. My left arm shook so much during the movement that the plastic cups almost always got knocked on the floor inside of twenty seconds. Without the ability to get them myself (and feeling utterly defeated), I simply let them lie there and resorted to tapping my finger from my nose to my ear.

Thankfully, Kirstin was there with me most of July 4th. She helped push me to do more exercises when I didn't want to, and around 4:00 p.m. she went out to get me the hot dog that had been promised to me before the surgery. I was very excited for this foolish and misguided treat, but my desire to feel normal and for brown mustard allowed me to press forward to a challenge that I probably should not have accepted.

There is nothing sexier than being awakened from an afternoon slumber to your wife holding a paper bag containing two mouthwatering processed meat snacks. I was excited for this meal. I had been looking forward to it all day, all week really. When those sauerkraut-covered dogs came out of the brown bag and were elegantly laid out upon my adjustable hospital tray, I almost wept tears of joy. As my wife generously, applied mustard to the dogs for us to cheers our country's birthday, I couldn't help but feel happy for this triumphant repast on the road to recovery. A hot dog on the 4th of July, brain surgery be damned.

This cavernous malformation might slow me down, but it wasn't going to take away my God-given rights as an American to shove processed meat snacks into my gullet. With the hot dog in my left hand and an iPhone in my right hand, I tried to snap a quick selfie. I missed my body in the frame of the first one. I tried again, but the second time the picture was too blurry. On the third attempt I really focused in on my right hand to get a full shot of myself eating the dog, but in my moment of intense focus, I must have dropped my hot dog onto the ground, because I got a great photo of me taking a bite out of air. When you can't feel a limb, it's hard to know where it is in space or what it's holding. Sadly, the five-second rule does not apply to hospital floors. Happily, my wife donated her hot dog to the patient and offered to snap a photo of me indulging in my American freedoms, this time using my right hand (see www.disconjugategaze.com).

Later that evening, Kirstin wheeled me into the visiting area to watch the fireworks along the East River. It was probably the best view I ever had for a fireworks display, but it was lost on me. All I could make out were intermittent flashes of different-colored light at varying intensities and distances. I couldn't make out any of the shapes, and because of my double vision, it appeared as if many of the explosions were taking place inside the hospital instead of over the river. I closed my eyes to avoid the dizzying display, hoping that in the darkness my wife wouldn't be able to tell the difference. Kirstin stood next to my wheelchair for the entire twenty-minute display, holding my hand and pretending that this was the most normal thing that two newlyweds could do on the 4th of July. Every once in a while, she would comment on how pretty it was and I would acknowledge her comment with a simple grunt or the standard "ohhh" or "ahhh." She knew I wasn't actually watching. I knew that she knew that I wasn't watching. But we both kept up the ruse. We continued to hold hands in the darkness of the hospital visiting room. We continued to hold hands and continued to pretend as if this situation was totally normal. We continued to hold hands together while we separately mourned the loss of our normal American future.

DAY 6: MOXIETIME!

Sundays are "off-days" at the rehabilitation center. Why, I do not know. I doubt it's a religious thing because a significant portion of the Upper East Side and the patients at this particular hospital are Jewish. It's probably a staffing decision made many years ago, but rehabbing from brain surgery shouldn't have off-days and, given that I was trapped in the hospital, I'd rather get some work done rather than sleep all day and watch *Alaskan Bush People*. But I digress.

Kirstin arrived around 11:00 a.m. with a cup of "outside" coffee that tasted excruciatingly bitter, but was infinitely better than what was available on the inside. Pre-surgery I was an avid coffee drinker. I wasn't a connoisseur, per se, but I drank two cups a day with regularity. One in the morning and one around 4:00 p.m. I preferred black iced coffee, and when I drank hot coffee it was ordered "dark" (with a splash of milk). In this immediate post-surgery time, my need for coffee had returned, but the way I took it changed. "Dark" coffee was too bitter for me. My palate had changed significantly. My taste buds had dulled considerably, and to consume the well-intentioned hospital food, I often had to add heavy amounts of salt, pepper, and contraband Tabasco. To my normally unmolested coffee, I added two to three teaspoons of sugar. The need to sweeten and season my food and drink was not a preference, but a requirement. That, coupled with my sedentary lifestyle and daily intake of steroids, helped me put on an unnecessary 30 pounds by the end of December, but that's a story for a different time.

After coffee and several rounds of eye exercises, my wife relayed that she thought it would be a good idea to get some fresh air and sunshine. I was concerned that we would get in trouble for leaving the hospital and cause a panic, but Kirstin responded: "What are they going to do? Arrest us?" A fair point, and one which I could not argue.

Still, I liked rules and insisted that we tell the nurses' station where we were going. I was nervous as we approached the station, but the head nurse barely looked up from her computer screen and simply said, "Okay." It was quiet on the rehab floor this Sunday and I don't think anyone wanted to make things harder. As Kirstin wheeled me through the main lobby, I tried to appear normal, but I felt like a teenager trying to sneak into an R-rated movie. Once we crossed the threshold of the building and into the fresh air, the sunlight was overwhelming. I had to shield my eyes with my good hand, even though I was already wearing a cheap pair of sunglasses. The natural light overwhelmed my system, and Kirstin stopped the chair a few feet outside of the hospital while I tried to collect myself.

"Can you see anything?" my wife asked hopefully. Her tone wasn't that of concerned partner, but of excited parent, though I couldn't tell why. I tried to pick my head up and look forward. Her tone indicated a surprise. Amid the white glow of light, I could subtly make out Kirstin's younger sister walking toward me. She was an amorphous smile bounding toward me, giving off a high-pitched "Hi" like she was holding keys to a new car.

As I tried to focus my gaze and say hello, something dropped in my lap. From where, I could not tell you, but after a few seconds I could tell what it was. It was Moxie! She wiggled in my lap and licked at my neck and face. It took a couple seconds longer before I could actually see her features or those of my sister-in-law, but when I was able to make out my surroundings I thanked Elka (my sister-in-law) and Kirstin repeatedly. Moxie kept right on bouncing in my lap and licking my face as she normally did when I came home from work. Our dog didn't notice any of my deficiencies and greeted me in just the same way that she always did.

Kirstin hugged me and said, "That's not my only surprise." A couple of minutes later, my college friend Steve walked up with a couple of processed-meat-filled sandwiches from my favorite deli. They wheeled me into the shade, and the five of us ate lunch outside in the ever-warming summer air. Normally a voracious eater of sandwiches, I probably finished a third of my "Italian Supreme" wrap, alternating bites for myself and scraps for the dog. Normally Kirstin would get on my case for feeding the dog human food, but today she let me spoil our furry companion. It was great to get some fresh air, to see my dog, and to eat some real food, but after about twenty minutes I felt overheated and asked to be wheeled back inside. Once back in my bed, I instantly fell asleep to happy dreams of soppressata and puppy licks.

DAY 7, 8, AND 9: NETFLIX, PODCASTS, AND OTHER WAYS TO PASS THE TIME

Having been in the hospital for over a week, the days started to blur together. Wake up, shower, go back to sleep, eat breakfast, head downstairs for OT, PT and speech. Return to room. Eat lunch, take a nap. Head downstairs for OT and PT, return to room. Take a nap.

I was much more alert in the second week, and my naps became shorter and shorter. To fill the extra time between sessions, I often watched a show on my iPad. To say that I "watched" programming is a bit of a misnomer, because at that time even on an 8x10-inch iPad at a distance of one foot, I couldn't totally make out the entire screen. In response to this issue, I mostly watched shows that I had already seen many times, like *The Simpsons* or *It's Always Sunny*. It was basically like an audiobook anyway, and I usually flipped the screen upside down after a couple minutes and just listened to the dialogue while I imagined the teleplay in my mind.

I also entertained myself by listening to podcasts. I'm quite certain I had never listened to a podcast prior to the surgery, and I don't listen to many now, but in the hospital, I avidly consumed them. My two favorite podcasts, *Serial* and *How Did This Get Made?* were about as different in terms of content and purpose as possible. *Serial* is a podcast the retells the story of an accused murderer and his trial through the voice of an investigative journalist. *How Did This Get Made?* is a podcast about the lunacy, extravagance, and implausibility of the poorly-written action movies guys like me watch incessantly. If I was feeling down after a difficult PT session, I'd turn to an over-the-top analysis of the scientific inaccuracies of the movie *Face Off.* If I felt like my intellect was wasting away, I would tune into *Serial* to see if the cell tower pings proved Adnan guilty or innocent.

I do often give thanks for having gone through this ordeal in the 21st century. Had I been diagnosed ten years earlier, there would not have been any podcasts to entertain me, no Netflix, and no Wi-Fi to distract from the monotony and sadness of a 17-day-long hospital stay. Had I been diagnosed twenty years earlier, the doctors would have used a far more invasive technique or not operated at all. Had I shown symptoms thirty years earlier, it's likely that the cavernous malformation would not have even been detected. I can't say with certainty that the cav-mal would have killed me were I born in 1960 rather than 1980, nor can I say that it would have killed me in the 21st century without surgical intervention. What I *can* tell you is that, were there ever an era to have your head cracked open for surgery, the 21st century is your best option.

DAY 10: SOME FEELING RETURNS

As I mentioned previously, the numbness that I felt prior to surgery was partial. I would say the sensation I felt on the outside of my limbs had been reduced to about 60% of normal by the cav-mal. But after the surgery, the numbness was absolute. I couldn't feel anything on the left half of my body. The increased numbness was expected by the surgeon, but it was terrifying. As with all surgeries of this kind, the results are fluid. That is to say, the surgeon *thought* there would be increased numbness and he *thought* it would subside, but it was impossible to predict. Nevertheless, with each passing day, the prospects of regaining sensation got worse and worse. By day ten, I was pretty concerned that I had opted in to a surgery that crippled me for life.

Even though the surgery did cripple me, it also (I believe) saved my life. When I get down about my deficiencies, I always try to remind myself to be thankful that I have a life at all. I still have reduced sensation on the left side of my body, but it is no longer absolute. I first felt something on the left side of my body when I was eating cereal that morning on day 10. At that time my facial muscles were a bit more compromised than they are today, and I often dribbled food and liquid at mealtimes. When some Cheerios dribbled out of my mouth and onto my arm, the feeling of smushed cereal and cold milk never felt so good. The partially consumed food didn't seem to carry any weight or texture, but it did feel cold. The absence of feeling is a hard thing to describe because in addition to not feeling the texture or pressure of an object, you also don't feel its relative heat or cold. Items have temperatures that often indicate something about them. Metal often feels cold and plastic often feels warm. Touch also has texture and pressure. With respect to movement, there is also spatial recognition and orientation. For the previous ten days, all of that was gone. If I closed my eyes and you bent my left toe, I couldn't tell you in which direction. If you held my hand, I couldn't tell if I was holding it back. The absence of feeling makes interacting with your surroundings very difficult. After I felt the milk and cereal on my arm, sensation began to return from the center of my body outward. The sensation I have today is far from complete, probably 30% of normal, but I'm grateful for every bit that I have. And it all started with some drooled cereal.

WEEKEND NUMBER TWO AND TERMINATOR GENISYS

Having been in the hospital for two full weeks, I was very lucky to have family and friends who would visit often. My wife came to visit daily and I cannot imagine the strength it must have taken for her to do that. To help her and to help me, she also called for basically all of my guy friends to come visit. Prior to the surgery, I had only told four people outside my family that I was having surgery. They were my friend Lindsey, a guidance counselor and the "ordained" minister at our wedding; my buddies Rob and Dave, both college friends and groomsmen in my wedding; and my head of school.

My male friends, mostly from college, visited often. They came in groups and brought greasy food, which I both appreciated and now lament, as I unknowingly gained twenty pounds in my three-week hospital stay. My college buddies and I have a tradition called "Bad Movie Night," whereby we get a pile of greasy food, some beers, and watch a bad movie together, *Mystery Science Theatre 3000*-style. Watching terrible movies is freeing because you can talk over them and no one will care. It's a great tradition that allows us to catch up on life without formalizing it. On the second Saturday in July, five of my college buddies descended on the hospital to watch *Terminator Genisys*.

(Spoiler alert: It is not a good film.)

The guys showed up around 7:00 p.m. with a couple of pizzas and garlic knots from a local pizzeria. The pizza, like the film, was not great, but it was better than steamed vegetables and pasta. I had reserved the visitors' room at the end of the floor for our "Bad Movie Night." As a screening room, this venue left much to be desired. The floor was linoleum, so every sound echoed in the sparsely-decorated room. All the tables and chairs were made of the same heavy fake wood, and they squeaked when moved. The back of each chair was padded with a plastic blue cushion. Though not aesthetically pleasing, the chairs were heavy (and thus unlikely to tip over) and simple (thus easy to clean). The television that I had "reserved" was mounted to the wall on the far end of the room and was probably about 20 inches diagonally. The closest I could get to the television in my wheelchair was about ten feet away, which was still well outside my field of vision. Given that my friends bought this bootleg version of the film on Grand Street, I wasn't the only one who couldn't see the picture clearly.

That night we sat around the table and I caught up on my friends' life events: new jobs, new apartments, different girlfriends, the Mets trading for Yoenis Cespedes. Eating pizza and talking about sports with my buddies on a Saturday night was such a simple sacrifice on their part, but it made all the difference in the world to me. I fell asleep less than 60 minutes in, but the guys stayed until the end, and I woke up to the surprisingly loud and bright credits. I had to re-watch the movie at home to confirm just how bad it was, and I still don't completely remember the plot of the film, but I do remember my friends giving up their Saturday night to feed me pizza and talk about life beyond the hospital.

DAYS 13, 14 & 15

The last couple of days in the hospital were tough. I had been indoors, save for one afternoon sandwich, for two weeks straight. I also had seen improvement in my mobility and stamina that made me think having 24-hour care was unnecessary. Feeling had started to return to the left side of my body, and I had convinced myself that it was just a waiting game until my body felt normal. That would never happen, and I was significantly deluded about my readiness to care for myself.

The last couple of days in the hospital focused on deliberate and important tasks I would need to relearn if I were to get around on my own. Though necessary, it was embarrassing to practice getting in and out of the bathtub (our apartment did not have a shower stall.) In occupational therapy we practiced brushing teeth standing up, cutting bread, and getting into and out of a fake car. The last activity was particularly difficult for me because I couldn't control my left arm and had to be careful not to sit on it.

My physical therapy also began taking on a more practical tone. We stopped focusing on balance and started focusing on using a walker properly and increasing the length of my walks. These walks took us all around the hospital and included short trips outside and into the heat. Though I tried not to show it, being out on the street was overwhelming. The hospital opened up to a relatively quiet circular driveway, but even there the combination of the heat and the moving vehicles was almost enough to knock me over. What I came to understand is that there is only so much you can accomplish in a closed environment. The real world isn't temperature-controlled with flat linoleum floors and overhead lighting. The real world can be hot or cold, can have cracked or uneven walkways, and people don't automatically get out of your way. That was a reality I had conveniently overlooked when assessing my own condition these past few weeks. Transitioning from the closed environment to an open environment was going to be hard, and my therapists were correct to push me to practice these life skills. I didn't accept my limitations or expect them to last long, but my last few days in the hospital tried to prepare me for the life of permanent disability that others knew I would have.

DAY 16: GOING HOME

I had gotten the go-ahead from the rehab doctor the day before, and all my appointments for Wednesday, July 15th had been cancelled. I was allowed to sleep in and skip the 5:00 a.m. shower so that I could tend to paperwork. And there was a lot of paperwork. There were all kinds of legal documents I needed to sign proving that I was choosing to leave the hospital. There were purchase orders I needed to sign for my walker and shower chair (to be delivered to our apartment.) And then there was the discharge packet, with all kinds of notes on what to expect when leaving the hospital. Lastly, there were a couple of pages listing all the medications I was taking. At this point there weren't too many. Most of the hard stuff had been discontinued within a week of the surgery, but I was still putting prescription ointment on my right eye, using saline drops ten times a day, taking a stool softener, and a blood thinner. Perhaps there were others, but I know that I was taking the blood thinner three times a day orally. I remember that because it was down from five times a day via stomach injection. My belly, which had quietly ballooned during my stay, was riddled with circular bruises the size of quarters.

Kirstin arrived around 11:00 that day to help me pack up the room. There was a surprising amount of stuff that I had accumulated over the past three weeks. Some of the items were medical, like the gauze pads that held my eye shut while I slept or the spirometer that I blew into to increase lung capacity after the surgery. Other items were gifts, like the mini-basketball hoops in which you can "shoot" the ping-pong ball toward the hoop by holding down a tiny catapult. Lastly, we had to pack up the clothing that I had been wearing.

I remember that it took a while for us to get the go-ahead to leave because there is a hospital rule that an orderly must push the wheelchair out of the building. I think it's a liability thing, so you can't sue the hospital if you fall while leaving, but whatever the case may be, it took a while for an orderly to become available. Kirstin and I took one last snooze together in the hospital bed while we waited.

"Daniel Ruf-er?" asked a voice entering the room.

"That's him," my wife replied, rubbing the sleep from her eye.

"You ready?" he asked.

"I sure am," I answered confidently before sitting up too quickly and getting light-headed.

"Slow down there, Daniel," the orderly said calmly. "There's no rush. Do you have his paperwork?" he asked, turning to my wife.

She retrieved it from the windowsill to the right of the bed and handed it to the muscular man in the white clothing. "He's just excited to get out of here."

"Oh, I bet, but we don't want you falling on the way out and ending up right back here. So, let's take it slow." I felt as if I was being condescended to, but the truth is I had to take it slowly because there was no other speed. As much as I wanted to jump out of bed and hurry out the door, anytime I sped up my movements my balance would be compromised, and I'd have to start all over. I had to take it slowly because that's the only speed I had anymore.

Eventually Kirstin and the nice orderly got me out of bed, into a wheelchair, down the elevator, through the lobby, out onto the street, and into a yellow taxi. All told it took about ten minutes and I didn't really do much of the work, but it was exhausting. I remember gleefully lowering the window to feel the rush of the hot summer air on my face as we pulled away from the hospital, but then I fell asleep, exhausted from the short journey from the hospital bed to the taxi. I don't remember exiting the taxi or entering our apartment, but I do remember waking up on the couch in the early afternoon to affectionate licks from Moxie.

DAY 1 (PART 2)

Thursday, July 16th began like most summer days for a teacher. I woke up after my wife had taken the dog out.

"Babe," she said from the living room. "I've got to go to work, but Moxie's been walked and I got you some breakfast." It was an iced coffee and croissant from a local bakery on the Upper West Side.

"Thanks," I responded from the bedroom while rolling over to a seated position with my feet on the ground. I wiped the sleep from the corner of my right eye and undid the tape that held it shut at night.

"Do you need help getting up?" she asked, entering the bedroom with a bouncy puppy right behind her.

"No, I think I got it, "I said, reaching for my tape-covered glasses. As I turned to my left, Kirstin swooped in and gave me a peck on the cheek.

"Don't do anything stupid while I'm at work." I nodded. "No showering on your own and no leaving the apartment without me or you mother." My mother was coming over to babysit me in an hour or two.

"Got it. Pinkie-swear," I said, extending my right hand.

She pushed it away. "You've got to use your left hand," she demanded. I tried to raise my limp left arm to meet hers, but all it did was jump back and forth like a mechanical arm trying to grasp a prize at the carnival. Kirstin caught my hand mid-shake and helped me complete the pinkie-swear. "Why don't you move to the couch while I'm still here. You can watch *SportsCenter!*"

Now she was speaking my language. I stood up by pushing off the bed with both hands and tried to steady myself as my left leg and hip forced me to rock back and forth. After a few seconds it calmed down, and Kirstin held my arm as we made the journey to the living room. Our NYC apartment was only 600 square feet, so this was not a long journey, but it probably took us about a minute to traverse the 15 feet from the bedroom to the couch. In in my defense, there were a lot of turns required to get there. My hospital room was quite large by comparison to our bedroom, and it had far less furniture. In our apartment, you needed to walk sideways to get from my side of the bed and past the dresser. Even before the surgery, I would often kick the dresser while walking to get in bed, so this was certainly going to be a problem area going forward. Kirstin was correct to help me on this maiden voyage.

Once on the couch, I collapsed into my favorite spot on the right side and Kirstin used the remote to turn the TV on and to ESPN. She pushed the coffee table closer so that I could reach the croissant and iced coffee. "Do you need anything before I go?" I shook my head no while suppressing the need to urinate. "Okay, remember, don't do anything stupid," she said with a forced smile. She blew me a kiss from across the room and said, "I love you," before turning down the hallway to the door.

"I love you too," I said with a mouthful of pastry. It was good to be home, but I quickly realized that my situation was no different than when I was in the hospital. I couldn't do anything or go anywhere on my own. The depressing state of affairs was further punctuated by a *SportsCenter* segment on a cancer patient's journey to meet his favorite hockey player. Why ESPN executives thinks the *SportsCenter* audience wants to see stories of sick children between baseball highlights I'll never know.

DAY 2 (PART 2): FLYING SQUIRRELS

My second day of freedom was punctuated by a trip to Central Park to watch my softball team against our hated rivals from National Bank. I was escorted by my buddy Ryan, formerly our first basemen during the glory days of the organization when we were known as F.W.B. (Friends with Benefits). As the years passed and our manager changed from a math teacher named Lauren to me, the team name changed immediately to Brews on First and finally to the glorious moniker Flying Squirrels. I'm not sure if it was the constant name changes or the emergence of two children in his family, but Ryan had since moved to Connecticut and retired from softball. So, when he agreed to chaperone me to the softball game it was a bit of a logistical sacrifice on his part, and I appreciated it greatly.

"Hey, Ryan," I said as he entered my apartment. I was seated on the coach with *Around the Horn* on the television. "Thanks for doing this."

"My pleasure," he said, scanning the room. "You look a lot better. There's more color in your face. It's good to see you, Mrs. Rufer," he said, referring to my mother, whose shift was about to end. "So, who are we playing today?"

"I think it's the assholes from National Bank, but you never know with the schedule." In our softball league, it was not uncommon to show up to a game only to find out that the team you were supposed to play wasn't there or you were on the wrong field or you were an hour early. Ultimately, it didn't really matter. The league was semi-competitive slow-pitch softball, and I was the team manager, pitcher, and lead-off hitter. Even though I couldn't play, I was very excited to be out there with my teammates and yell nonsensical statements of support into the warm summer air.

"Should we get going?" Ryan asked me.

"Sure," I replied. "I've just got to get my shoes and ankle brace on before we go." I always wore one knee-high sock on my left leg when I played softball so that I would have a layer between the ankle brace and my skin. Even though I wasn't playing, I thought it important to get in uniform.

"I'll go grab that for you," my mother offered, walking back into the bedroom to retrieve the socks and the brace.

"They should be in the top right dresser drawer," I replied.

My mother returned with one bright red sock and one black lace-up ankle brace, which didn't match my light-blue mesh shorts, white t-shirt jersey, black hat, and black sneakers. I like to think that my utter lack of coordinated dress distracted hitters, but I don't have the statistics to prove it. My mother placed the sock and brace on the arm of the sofa to my right. I reached for my left leg with both of my arms and pulled it over my right leg slowly and inefficiently.

"Do you want help?" my mother asked.

"Nope. I can do this myself." Both Ryan and my mother backed away slightly to give me some space. As I reached for the sock, my left leg fell off my right leg and back to the floor with a thud. Both spectators lunged forward to help. "I've got it," I said displaying a bravado externally that I did not have internally. I pulled my leg back up over my right knee and started to pull the giant red sock into place. Once that was accomplished, I pulled the ankle brace over my foot and pushed my leg away while holding the upper part of the brace. My grip on the brace slipped and my leg went smashing into the coffee table.

"Are you okay?" they both asked. I was. It probably should have hurt, but I didn't have enough sensation in my leg at that time to feel pain. The second time I pushed my leg away to bring the brace into position, it worked. Then I began the arduous task of tightening the laces. I could feel their eyes on me wanting to help, but they politely diverted their gaze whenever I would look up, and allowed me to continue.

After a minute or two of struggling with a total lack of strength in my left hand and the shakiness of the arm itself, I slumped back into the sofa, exhausted from my efforts. I took a moment to catch my breath and said, "Mom, can you help me with the shoes?" She obliged and completed the task in less than half the time it took me to lace up the brace.

When she was done, I leaned into the arm of the couch on my right side and pushed off with my upper body to stand. I took a second or two to balance myself and allow my left leg to stop shaking. Then I stepped forward a few paces to the dining table and put on my half-taped sunglasses. "I'm ready if you are," I said, turning to face Ryan. He walked across the room, grabbed the walker from its stowed position, and pushed it so that it was right in front of me. He stood in front of the walker, blocking it from sliding forward, and I positioned my hands on the handle bars. "Bye, mom. Please lock the door when you leave."

I could tell that she wanted to hug me, but then didn't because of how juvenile this whole episode was making me feel. Instead, she just said, "I love you. Be careful," as if we were two adolescents about to ride our bikes to the playground.

I shuffled down the interior hallway and into the elevator with Ryan spotting me the entire way. Once we got out onto the sidewalk, I motioned to Ryan that needed a moment. The heat, brightness, and noise of the city in July was overwhelming. I felt flushed, weak, and unsteady all at the same time. It took about thirty seconds for that light-headed feeling to subside before we began the one-block walk to the park.

This exact walk to Central Park was what I used to complete every morning to get to the subway. Pre-surgery, I could walk from the front door of my apartment building to the train platform in five minutes. On this day, it took three times as long. Because of the heat and the brightness, I held my gaze downward and shuffled my feet so that my good leg always maintained contact with the sidewalk. It was good that we started early, because it took us a similar amount of time to walk the concrete path from the entrance of the park to the field.

Upon arrival to the field, I could see many of my teammates on the park-bench dugout changing out of their work clothes and into our totally mismatched t-shirt and shorts uniform. Those who were wearing shoes came over to greet me with excitement, smiles, and a little bit of fear. About half of my teammates had visited me in the hospital and I had downplayed the severity of my injuries in email correspondence so it must have been striking to see their team manager arrive using a walker. As they encircled me and patted me on the shoulder I became overstimulated, and Ryan stepped in to help me to the bench. Over the next month or two, I would often struggle with overstimulation, and I was thankful that Ryan was there to recognize it and get me seated before I fainted.

After a moment, my buddy Dave came over and smacked the brim of my cap a little too hard. "What's up, Dan? Do you have the line-up? We're going to start in a couple of minutes." Dave had taken over pitching and managerial duties while I was in the hospital and was kindly offering me the opportunity to resume my role.

"If you write it out, I'll read it," I said to him.

"Done," he exclaimed before running back in to the field to hear the ground rules from the umpire. While he was away, I perused his lineup card and made a few changes. When he returned, I showed it to him. He laughed and said "Alright, read it, boss." I tried to rise to meet the team as Dave called everyone in for the line-up, but I lost my balance and fell back to the bench. Seeing this Dave called for everyone to come into the dugout, where I proceeded to read out the line-up.

"Batting first and pitching, Dave."

"Batting second and playing second, Karen."

I read out all ten players on the line-up card and with all my might raised my right hand above my head for our ceremonial pre-game chant. I softly yelled: "One, two, three, squir-rels!" and the rest of the team then yelled "Go nuts." It's prob-ably the best chant in all mixed-gender recreational softball, and it felt good to say it once again. Our team took the field and a player from their team walked out to the batter's box. He wasn't from National Bank, and I don't remember much more of the game, but I do remember the immense feeling of belonging that was lacking from my life in the hospital. Whether we won or lost I couldn't tell, but I will always remember that evening as one step in the right direction toward regaining a sense of normalcy in my life.

JULY AND AUGUST

The rest of the summer was hard. Every Monday, Wednesday, and Friday I took a taxi to the hospital for physical therapy and occupational therapy. On days that I didn't have therapy, I was home performing my exercises (balancing on one foot, turning cards with my left hand, reading letters off an eye chart, sorting coins, forcing smiles, etc.). It was monotonous and bore few results. It was also isolating and sad. Because I was well enough to go to the bathroom by myself and because my wife had to work, I was often at home (alone) with my thoughts all day long. Outwardly I tried to project that everything was okay, but the little progress I made took its toll on me mentally. My wife recounts my time in the hospital as the hardest part of the whole ordeal, but for me it was the six weeks at the end of the summer, when I was often left alone to contemplate my deficiencies.

Thankfully, I had a little furry animal to keep me company. I also had a neighbor who kindly volunteered to take me on walks every Tuesday and Thursday. Her name was Betty and she was a retired divorcee in her late fifties. Like us, she was a dog owner, and we had known her fairly well prior to my surgery. While I was in the hospital she was kind to Kirstin and the two of them often shared a glass of wine after Kirstin returned home from the hospital. Also, she generously walked Moxie on days when Kirstin came home late. Upon my return from the hospital, she offered to help in any way that she could. I replied that I too needed to be walked every day, and would she consider keeping me company? She obliged and the two of us shared walks on every Tuesday and Thursday for the rest of the summer.

Our walks started out small, just to the end of the block and back. I was using the walker for the majority of this time. Staying on avenues and main streets was important because that's where the better sidewalks are. As I got stronger, we would venture further and further away from the apartment. We'd usually walk up Columbus because there was less human traffic and more of the corners had inclines that were easier to navigate. As we walked, she would tell me about her children--a son living in China, engaged to be married in less than a year, and a daughter "figuring it out" in California. I was intensely focused on not tipping over, so I didn't add much to the conversation, but I think as much as I needed someone to walk me, she needed someone to talk to. Our journeys never went very far, but it was a breakthrough when we both felt comfortable enough to venture into Central Park. Navigating a walker over anything other than flat surfaces is hard. Traversing the brickwork that surrounds Central Park is even harder; the front wheels of the walker often caught on the seams, and it took a light touch to clear them. Our walks kept increasing in distance and duration, and I always needed a nap when they were finished.

In the later part of the summer I ditched the walker and started using a cane. The distances I could travel shrank once again to a few blocks, but Betty was there to chaperone me. Over time, we were able to extend the time and distance of our walks once again. By late August, I was able to make it all the way around the reservoir (1.6 miles in circumference). I had hoped that by then I would be rid of the cane, but that was not meant to be. In retrospect, that should have been enough information for me to take time off from work, but I was bored and lonely and I didn't like the idea of anyone else doing my job for me. So, I returned to work just eleven weeks after the surgery on Thursday, August 27th.

DEANS' MEETING

In the weeks and months that followed my surgery, there were many first meetings. Many of my friends (though not all) had seen me either in the hospital or in the intervening six weeks of recovery at home. Most of my colleagues did not know about my condition or ensuing surgery. The ones who did, the administrative team plus one or two others, received this email on July 7th:

Colleagues,

George, Hugo and Arvind already know this, but I asked them to keep it quiet for a couple of days whole I was healing and figuring out what the recovery would be like.

As it turns out the numbness thing that I was dealing with in my left leg had nothing to do with my back and everything to do with some malformed blood vessels on my brain stem. The good need is that I had symptoms that alerted me this health risk. The bad news is that to alleviate the problem I underwent brain surgery on June 25th and I've been in the hospital recovering ever since. I am currently at a rehab facility on the upper east side and I will be until next Wednesday (my estimated discharge date).

The recovery is a very long process, but the good news is that II am on the mend and everyone of really happy with my progress. By the time school starts the only thing that will be noticeable should be a lazy right eye and some news glasses.

I didn't mean to keep this for all of you, but I also didn't want to worry snuone too much since when it was first discovered We did not think brain surgery was going to necessary.

If you want to contact Me please use my personal email address at xxxx@gmail.com or 917-555-xxxx.

George, Hugo, and Arvind have a few more details in case this email is as littered with typos as I think it, but the bottom line is that I An on the mend and will be operating at near 100^ by the time the school year starts.

I will do my best to respond to personal emails and trxts, but until I get a functioning pair of glasses II will not be responding to this email address. My auto-response will be changed tomorrow.

This is not a secret, but I am not emailing any kids or parents with this information. And I would appreciate it if we could keep this need in adult circles for the time being.

All the best,

Dan

Ps I suffered no cognitive impairment as a result of this surgery. All of the typos in this email are compliments of an iPhone and done newly terrible eyesight. If I ever made fun of one of for warring glasses? I deeply apologize. Life without perfect vision is really really hsrd.

So, Thursday, August 27th was a big day. It was the first time I had gone to work since mid-June and would be the first time I would see many of my work colleagues. While I had ditched the walker, I was still heavily reliant on a cane, and my glasses consisted of safety goggles with surgical tape over the right lens. I was hunched over like an old man when I walked and I was physically quite weak. Truthfully, I shouldn't have been there, but I made it a point to return to normalcy, so I returned to work on time for the very first administrative meeting of the year.

I tried to get there early to avoid the awkwardness of walking into a full room, but my taxi got caught in summer traffic and I was simply on time rather than twenty minutes early, as I had planned. The classroom where the meeting was being held was half-full when I arrived. Those that were in it were swapping stories about the summer and expressing immodest regret at having to return to work. The door was open when I reached the threshold, and I shuffled to the first open chair to avoid displaying my weakened state through my jerky, unsteady walking.

Kim jumped up to pull out the chair for me as I tried to get seated.

"Thank you," I uttered, keeping my gaze down toward the floor.

"Welcome back, Dan," Ilana said. "I'm so happy that you are okay."

Arvind chimed in by saying, "You look good." I knew that I didn't, but I appreciated the pleasantries nonetheless.

"How about that *Walking Dead* episode last Sunday?" I asked, trying to deflect the tension in the room even though I hadn't seen the show.

None of the three took the bait. "We're really glad that you are here," Arvind said. "We're glad that you are okay."

"Thanks," I said looking up sheepishly, but before I could get anything else out, three more administrators entered the room.

"Hello everybody," said the head of school joyfully as he entered the room and took his seat at the head of the table. "Welcome back. You all look tan and rested." He paused. "Except for Dan, but he had brain surgery, so we'll give him a pass." I appreciated the joke at my expense, but the others in the room cringed. "We're waiting for a couple more people to start, but if you check your inbox, you will find an email with Hugo's agenda for today."

FACULTY
ORIENTATION

The administrative meeting was relatively uneventful from there on out, and I was happy to have it behind me. As nervous as I was to return to work, I felt fortunate that it was a slow roll-out. First, I met with the faculty that knew of my surgery, the then faculty that didn't know, and last with the kids. Faculty orientation was on Monday, August 31st, three days after the administrative meeting. I was nervous. How would my colleagues react to seeing me in this weakened state? Would they pity me? Would they be scared of me? Would they be angry with me for keeping this a secret? To be honest, I got a little bit of all of these reactions, but mostly I got support and smiles, just as I would have after any other summer break.

I arrived at work about twenty minutes before the meeting was supposed to start, but this being a school, many faculty members (particularly the longtime ones) were already there drinking coffee and swapping summer stories. The meeting took place in the gym because it was the only room that could hold all of us. Foldable tables and plastic chairs were set in rows and columns all throughout the gym. Most chairs were empty, but some had backpacks and other bags that marked territory for the meeting. The nervous side of me expected everyone to turn and stare at me in hushed silence upon arrival, but that didn't happen. Instead, I quietly opened the door and walked in. No one noticed. I took this opportunity to shuffle over to the corner table nearest to the entrance and take a seat. My gaze was downward while I took off my backpack and placed it on a chair.

As I started to pull out a second chair and affix my cane to the side of the table, I was startled by a pat on the back and a loud "Rufer, how you been?" It was Chante, a boisterous physical education teacher from the lower school. She and I played softball together and often hung out at the beach in the summer, but for obvious reasons I hadn't seen her since June. I turned my head to the right to meet her gaze and I could see her happy smile turn to concern and shock.

"Give me a second," I said, placing my cane on the chair to the right. Chante helped me push in the chair that held the cane and then took the seat directly across from me.

"Are you okay?"

"Yes... No... Sort of... It's a long story." I paused, wanting to answer her questions, but not wanting to recount all the details. Chante, sensing that I was about to reveal something serious, asked if she could get me a coffee or something else to drink. I replied: "A water would be great."

"You got it. I'll be right back." I lowered my head while she was away, trying to be invisible to the steadily increasing crowd emerging from the entranceway. Most of the arriving teachers instinctively walked to the breakfast bar for coffee, but a few of my high school colleagues noticed me sitting in the corner and came over to say hi. Like Chante, they had looks of concern and surprise in their faces when I looked up to reveal my taped-over safety goggles. I had started to explain what happened when Chante came back with a cup of water and sat down. When I took a sip, the other three sat down as well.

"Remember when I was having those back issues last spring?" Even though I had two months to practice, I wasn't particularly good at telling this story. It was emotional for me, and outside of the medical profession pretty much nobody knew what a cavernous malformation was. So typically, I just told people that I had a brain tumor and that while it got removed and I was going to be okay, there was still considerable damage done to my left side of my body and right side of my face, including my right eye. Most people wanted to know if I was going to get better. I usually said that the mobility stuff should resolve itself in a few months, but the facial stuff was likely permanent. That was usually enough to elicit sympathy and a half-hearted "Well, you look good" statement. But every once in a while, someone would want to know more. One of these nosy nellies was in this initial group. He was a biology teacher, so his interest may have been based in pure inquiry, but it was uncomfortable nonetheless.

"So, can they do a surgery to fix your face?" Before I could answer, he added: "Isn't there a realignment surgery they can do with the eye? My nephew had a realignment surgery last spring. I could get you the doctor's information," he said while pulling out his phone.

"Well--" I responded.

He cut me off again before I could finish. "Dr. Johnson is his name. I could email it to you."

Chante, sensing my discomfort, jumped in to say, "Slow down, Bill, give him a chance to answer."

"Well," I paused. "There is a surgery they can do to realign my right eye, but it probably will just be cosmetic." I pulled up my glasses to show my inward-pointing and relatively immobile right eye. "It's unlikely that the doctors can get the two eyes working together again, but it should look better for pictures." Bill started to ask another question, but this time I jumped in. "Also, they don't want to do any surgery for a least a year, to see where these things settle." That seemed to satisfy Bill for the moment.

By then most of the faculty had found seats around the room. My table had two open seats, one at each end, but nobody was looking our way. As the head of school tapped on the microphone in an effort to quiet the buzz in the room, I motioned for the four sitting at my table to come in closer. "Guys, if you don't mind, do you think you could pass this information about me along? I don't really want to retell this 120 times today." The group responded with nods of agreement as my boss started in on his annual "welcome back" speech.

As he continued on about what a great year it was going to be, peppering in sports metaphors like "knock it out of the park" every few minutes, two more adults joined our table. The first was a lower school teacher who used a walker to get around because of a hip injury. The second was a high school computer teacher who was recovering from triple-bypass surgery. It was strange, but somewhat poetic that all the injured faculty had found themselves in this corner of the gym. To be fair, the meeting had started and these were among the only seats available. Even though it initially made me feel sad that I was sitting at some sort of self-appointed invalid table, I came to appreciate my conversations with these two colleagues, because they knew what it was like to lose your mobility.

When the meeting broke, most of the faculty left the gym for a team-building scavenger hunt at Grand Central Station. Margaret of the injured hip, Steve of the repaired heart, and I stayed back. The assistant head of school came over and offered to get us a taxi if we wanted to go on the excursion. I was about to say yes, when Margaret said, "We're good." I'm glad she did, because by the time Steve and I walked from the gym to the high school offices, I was exhausted. I sat down on the two-seat couch in my office, put my head on a pillow, and fell asleep in the air-conditioned confines until it was time for lunch. The rest of the day is a blur, but it was good to be back on campus with colleagues who cared about me and doing work about which I cared.

STUDENT ORIENTATION

The third and in many ways most daunting step in my reintroduction to work occurred with the students on Wednesday, September 9th. I'm generally amazed with how kids deal with change, and I trusted that this group of kids would welcome me back with open arms. But the teenager is a strange animal. I didn't think they would make fun of me, the way I looked, or the pronounced lisp in my speech, but I was concerned that they might be scared of me. Would they shy away from me as if I were a hideous monster? The teenagers I teach are not the raunchy teens of a John Hughes movie; the teenagers I teach are sophisticated, have already traveled the world, and know the purpose of a demitasse cup. They aren't perfect, but they generally have good manners, and I had a good relationship with the group. Still, I was extremely nervous to see them on student orientation. As the grade dean, I was supposed to have it together. I was supposed to be organized and command authority. Would they respect me when they saw that I couldn't walk in a straight line? Would they laugh when I had trouble pronouncing words that began with the letter "f"? Would they look away when my taped-over glasses became too much of a distraction? I was nervous for all these reasons, but I had committed a long time ago to this group and to myself. I wasn't going to let a small thing like brain surgery get in the way of finishing my job. So, on the 9th of September, I put on my khakis, hopped in a taxi, and headed downtown to reintroduce myself to the Class of 2018.

I greeted the sophomore class at the front door and instructed them to head toward the auditorium for an assembly. As they entered the reactions were mostly subdued and teenagerly.

"Hi, Mr. Rufer."

"Happy fall, Mr. Rufer."

"Where do we go?"

"What happened to your eye?"

I had sent an email home with a brief synopsis of my health struggles, but I knew that many of them didn't read it. That was okay. I expected it. And, like any good educator, I planned a presentation.

Once a critical mass of students had arrived, the other adults and I shooed them into the auditorium and out of the bathroom, hallways, and other places teenagers linger. Most had taken their seats as I lumbered and limped down the center aisle. Once I made it to the front of the auditorium where the first slide of my PowerPoint, entitled "Welcome Back, Sophomores!" was being displayed, I turned to face the group. I took a deep breath and asked for quiet. To my relief, they mostly complied.

"Welcome back, Class of 2018. You are now sophomores." Sarcastic clapping and hollers erupted from the boys before the girls quieted them with their disdainful glances. "As you can see, I went through a bit of a health scare this summer.' I paused, trying to remain confident. "But I'm okay now. The back issue I had last spring turned out not to be a back issue at all, but a tiny ruptured blood vessel in my brain. To prevent it from getting worse, the doctors had to perform surgery. In the process they had to sever two nerves, one that controls my right eye and one that controls the right side of my face. I have a slide that shows exactly where the surgery took place." I clicked to a slide entitled "My Summer Brain Surgery." It looked like this:

- Not a back injury (cavernous malformation)
  - Cavernous malformations are clusters of abnormal, tiny blood vessels, and larger, stretched-out, thin-walled blood vessels filled with blood in

the brain. These blood vessel malformations can also occur in the spinal cord, the covering of the brain (dura), or the nerves of the skull. Cavernous malformations range in size from less than one-quarter inch to 3-4 inches. (AANS, 2008)

o   Discovered in April. Doubled in size by June. And needed to be excised.

o   Originally pressing on the nerves that control sensation in my leg. When it grew, I lost sensation in my arm, trunk, neck, ear, and heard a constant ringing (tinnitus).

I read the bullet points and elaborated on them like as I would a typical PowerPoint presentation. Then I flipped to a slide showing a lateral view of the brain and pointed with a laser to the location of the cavernous malformation. Next, I turned to a slide of the posterior view of the brain and described how the doctor pulled the two hemispheres of my brain apart, severing two cranial nerves in the process before stitching me back up.

"And that's what I did this summer," I said before looking back at the audience. "Any questions?"

The room was silent. It may have been the most silent group of teenagers in the history of mankind. I thought they would be relieved if they knew the details of the surgery, but instead they just blankly stared back at me. I had made it way less comfortable.

Realizing my mistake, I clicked to the next slide and said, "Okay, let's take a look at what we have planned for the rest of the day." In retrospect, it was not the best way to describe a life-altering experience, but it's what happened, and now they had most of the answers to the questions that they didn't know they had.

I dismissed the students from the auditorium to embark on the various orientation activities. Once they were gone, I went back to my office and thought about that interaction and how I might make thing more comfortable going forward.

Several hours later, after all the fall schedules were distributed, lockers were assigned, and textbooks downloaded, I called for one final meeting in the auditorium. When the students settled in, I clicked on the new presentation I had just created, entitled: "How You Can Help Me."

- You can help me out by
  - answering questions of inquisitive students so I don't have to answer them
  - picking up your jackets, cleats, etc.
  - not sneaking up on me
  - not jumping on me
  - offering to hold doors
  - offering to carry stuff

This time I got a few chuckles and a few offers to carry my laptop back to my office. I got a few hugs from the more sensitive students, and firm handshakes from some of the ne'er-do-well boys. The second part of the orientation went about as well as I could have imagined, and the heavy-lifting of telling students about my surgery was basically over.

FIRST DAY OF CLASSES

The first day of academic classes was what I perceived as one of the final benchmarks on the road to recovery. I still view it as a major benchmark, but one at the beginning of my recovery. Nevertheless, it was a big day. Because I was a grade dean, I taught a half load, equal to two Algebra 2 classes, so that I was free to troubleshoot class of 2018 issues, ranging from broken lockers to tragic breakups to ailing parents and everything in between. On this first day of academic classes only one of my sections met, but it was first period.

When I walked into the room, I was pleased to see some familiar faces. About half of the students were 10th graders who knew of my surgery and understand my newfound disabilities. The other half were 11th graders, some of whom I had taught in middle school, and all of whom were sitting quietly, waiting for me to speak. It was uncharacteristically quiet for a room full of teenagers. I could tell that they were nervous to see how this was going to play out.

"By your silence, I can see that many of you have heard of my health struggles. In the 10th grade orientation I explained my situation fully, but it seemed to scare everyone, so I'm not going to do that now. I had brain surgery. My right eye doesn't work, my face is paralyzed, and left side of my body is numb. If you have any questions, you can ask Eduardo." Eduardo was a precocious but kind young man that I'd taught in 6th, 8th, and now 10th grade. Even though Eduardo shifted in his seat and flushed with anxiety, he would be up to the challenge. I paused for a moment and pulled out a stack of papers. "Take one and pass it back," I said, distributing my standard day-one "syllabus and course expectations." Once everyone had a paper, I looked at my roster and called on a random student to begin reading. It wasn't the most elegant way to start a class, but it was far more efficient, and by this time the next day everyone who needed to know of my surgery would know. It was a relief not to keep my health a secret anymore.

As much as the physical recovery from an event like this taxes your body, the emotional drain is just as severe. Right or wrong, I felt I had to manage people's expectations and reactions. I didn't want my illness to be their problem or a source of anxiety for them. I didn't want people to view me as anything less than I was, and so I carefully controlled the flow of information. That's probably not the best course of action for someone going through a similar ordeal, but it's how I approached the information issue, and now it was basically over.

When the class ended, I quickly shuffled to the bathroom and threw up. When I had steadied myself, I took the elevator down to the nurse's office and fell asleep for nearly two hours.

CHAPEL TALK

One of the first people to seek me out upon my return to campus was our school chaplain. Though I don't consider myself to be particularly religious, Rev is a kind and caring man, and I enjoy talking with him. In addition to my own talk therapist, I leaned heavily on Reverend Hummel to get me through the first few weeks of school. Once I had my footing at work, he asked if I might be willing to address the high school at one of our weekly chapels. I agreed, and below is the transcript of the speech that I gave on Thursday, October 8th:

Chapel Talk- Rufer

Among the bevy of things I have tried since undergoing surgery are: talk therapy, physical therapy, occupational therapy, speech therapy, swimming, writing, meditating, praying, and delivering a chapel speech. There is no one way to heal from an injury-- or any kind of loss, for that matter. For the sake of this speech, I will pinpoint the beginning of my healing process as the moment that I awoke from surgery late in the afternoon on Thursday, June 25th, 2015.

Whether as a goof or in all seriousness, I received a book from the Schmidt advisory on the second day of school, entitled The 12 Stages of Healing. *The gift cost $1 and earned their advisory 10 points in the Class of 2018 scavenger hunt. They probably would have won if they had turned in all their photos, but they can rejoice in the fact that they gave me a book that I actually read. Like most self-help books purporting to offer a pathway with which to deal with an emotional, physical, or other type of crisis, there were some parts of this book that I liked and others that I merely glossed over. For the sake of this chapel talk and for* *my own understanding of the healing process, I have distilled Dr. Epstein's 12 stages down to five. They are not meant to be linear and they're not meant to be exclusive, but I think I can use these five stages to talk about my healing process and perhaps impart some knowledge to all of you here. The five stages I refer to in this speech are:*

1. *Suffering*
2. *Stuck in perspective*
3. *Reclaiming my power*
4. *Acceptance*
5. *Community.*

Stage 1: Suffering.
Those of you who are paying attention in your philosophy and religion classes will know that suffering is one of the four noble truths bestowed upon us by the Buddha. When he was writing about suffering, I don't think he meant getting a hole drilled in your head and spending three weeks in the hospital learning how to walk again. But I think it applies nonetheless. Without hitting bottom, how would you know which way is up? How can I appreciate the beautiful complexity of the human brain without first understanding how completely wrong things can go? For those of you who can walk freely without assistance, that in and of itself is a miracle. I'm not trying to make anyone feel guilty, but cut one tiny wire, one nerve ending in the base of your brain, and all that goes away. For those of you who can see freely without the assistance of contact lenses or glasses or surgery, that too is a miracle. Cut one tiny wire in the base of your brain and, to paraphrase Zoolander, I "can only see left". Given all the tens of thousands or millions of neural connections that exist within the brain, it is a miracle that most of us are walking around and seeing as well as we can. Did I need to go through this ordeal to appreciate the complexity of the human brain? Probably not. But if you think that I will for even one second take for granted the ability to walk freely or see without glasses when I am healed, you are sorely mistaken. Suffering is as necessary for growth as it is for understanding.

Stage 2: Stuck in perspective.
I moved into the second stage of healing when I was discharged from the regular hospital and moved to the rehabilitation floor. You might think that waking up from surgery with a completely

paralyzed face, completely numb left leg and arm, and two eyes that could not focus was the low point, but being moved to the rehab floor was actually the worst. As the surgery and recovery was explained to me, I thought I would be out of the hospital in five to seven days. After five days on various medical floors, I was cleared to move to the rehab floor. There I was told I would need to stay in the hospital for an additional two to three weeks. This was devastating. As much as I was suffering in the ICU, I just kept thinking, this is only going to be for about a week, then I'll be fine and I can go home. *I didn't know how these parts of my body were going to start working again in five to seven days, but that was my expectation. Once that didn't come true, I began to wonder if I would ever heal properly. For that first week on the rehab floor I couldn't let go of my anger at still being in the hospital. I was angry at the doctor for lying to me and I was angry at my body for betraying me. It took me a good two weeks of living with the profound changes to my body to truly accept the seriousness of my situation. I eventually accepted that the physical healing process will take between six to twelve months and may never be complete. Once I made that statement to myself, once I let go of my pre-surgery expectations, my mood lightened, and I actually began to heal faster.*

Stage 3: Reclaiming my power.
It's easy to feel helpless when you are suffering. It's easy to feel helpless when you feel powerless. It's easy to feel helpless when you can't do for yourself. The physical therapists at the hospital knew this acutely. A couple days after I got to the rehab floor, an 85-year-old man came in after a massive stroke. He couldn't walk, he couldn't talk, and he could really only move his hands enough to put a pill cup to his mouth. From the conversations I overheard in the therapy room, he seemed to have lived a very full life prior to the stroke. Right now, he was barely moving. One day, his wife came in pleading with the therapist to help him along. They asked her what it was that he liked to do. She replied, "Well, he's a really great water skier." It was hard to believe that this 85-year-old man, confined to a chair with movement capabilities of his arm reduced to about 10 inches, water-skied frequently on the weekends with his grandchildren. I didn't think too much of the conversation after I left, but there was a palpable excitement in the therapy gym by the time I got

there the next day. A few minutes later, the man's wife returned with a water ski rope. With his wife cheering him on and about four staff members supporting him, the therapist recreated the experience of standing up on water skis for this man. How much was really him standing up out of his chair and leaning back into the rope, I have no idea. But I do know is that for that short moment, those therapists gave him back his power, gave him back his hope, and he smiled as big of a smile as he could possibly muster. So, did I. I'm not going to tell you that he was doing cartwheels down the hallway the next day. That just isn't true, but I do know that by the time left he was using a walker, which by itself seemed very unlikely just a few days earlier. Sometimes you can't reclaim your power on your own; you need a little help. He got that from his wife and a water ski rope. I got mine from a beach ball and a whiffle ball bat.

Stage 4: Acceptance.
The process of reaching acceptance is one that, for me, was iterative in nature. That is to say, I had to do it many different times, for different things, and in different ways. First, I had to accept that nothing was wrong with my leg. I had to accept that the cause of my malfunctioning limb was actually something wrong with the nerve endings deep in my brain. I had to accept that brain surgery was the only thing that could stop this from worsening. I had to accept that in order for this to get better, the doctors had to damage some of the working parts of the rest of my body. Then I had to accept that my time in the hospital would be far longer than anticipated. Then I had to accept that I was going to need a walker for a certain amount of time. Then I had to accept that I couldn't go on the street by myself for a few weeks. And, most recently, I had to accept that teaching was going to be tiring. Very tiring. And that I would have to plan to be indoors by 8:00 and in bed by 9:00 every night. Acceptance is an integral part of the healing process. It allows you to relieve mental pressure on your own expectations.

Stage 5: Community.
This is where you all come in. I had a community helping me in the hospital. There was my wife and her family, my parents, my college buddies, and the select few that I told of my condition here at Grace. But I knew that the only way I could ever feel close to whole was if I was able to return to work. That said, there was

127

never a question in my mind as to whether I would return this September. During the opening faculty days, several of my colleagues asked me, "Didn't you ever consider taking the year off?" No, not for a second. This is where I want to be and this is the place that I knew would make me feel whole. I may not be able to tap dance yet or use the patented Mr. Rufer two-marker technique at the whiteboard just yet, but I'm here. Being here doing what I love with people that I care about makes me feel more healed than any balancing exercise I had to do (ad nauseum) in the hospital.

So why am I telling you this story? This is not the story I had planned to tell. When Reverend Hummell and I spoke in the spring, he and I discussed the possibility of me giving a chapel talk. It revolved around my relationship with my younger sister, Katie. She is developmentally disabled and lives in a group home here in Manhattan. It was to be a story of compassion, empathy, and life perspective. But so is this. What I meant to share with you was that, through my relationship with my sister, I had a unique perspective on the way the world works. Most of us can't understand the difficulties that the disabled experience every day as they go about their lives. But if you live with someone who is disabled, or work with someone who is disabled, or befriend someone who is disabled, you can certainly empathize with the hurt that they at times feel in a world that wasn't made for them or stuck in a body that doesn't function well in this world. Unfortunately for me, I can both empathize and sympathize. The motor skills I have on the left side of my body are almost identical to what my sister can muster throughout her entire body. A phrase often said in my family: "It could be worse."

So, you're smart enough to ask again, what's the point, Mr. Rufer? The point is to understand that while it could be worse, that doesn't mean that you can't make it better. You can do the simple things like offer a hand or a seat to someone who is need. You can keep the hallway clear so that a bumbling teacher can make his way around the second floor to play his own personal game of "I Spy" with track pants, sweatpants, and ripped jeans as the target. You can give a smile to someone who is hurting or without prompting simply ask how someone is feeling. You can do all that, and you can count your blessings, as I do every day.

Thank goodness I live in New York with the best hospitals in the entire world.

Thank goodness both my family and my wife's family live nearby.

Thank goodness for the perfect group of friends who were willing to come visit me in the hospital despite their noticeable discomfort.

Thank goodness I had my operation in the summer. If there was snow on the ground, I'd be housebound.

Thank goodness for elevators.

Thank goodness for Darrelle Revis and Yoenis Cespedes for lifting my spirits and carrying my sports teams to new heights.

Thank goodness for all of your kindness and attention these past few months.

And thank you for listening to me speak these last minutes.

INTIMACY

For the first eight weeks after I was discharged from the hospital, I threw up once a day, either before work in my own bathroom or at work in the faculty bathroom in the basement. Most of the time my urge to vomit came with the first thing I ate each day. It was weird. I wasn't nauseous when I woke up, but something about the smell of food triggered a gag reflex in me. And not all day, but just in the morning. The surgery that was performed also slightly damaged my sense of smell and taste, though I think that has largely returned to normal. For the first eight weeks out of the hospital, I threw up once a day and pretty consistently took a two-hour nap. All of this is to say that I wasn't particularly interested in sex.

To be fair I don't think my wife was interested in sex either but, come our anniversary on October 18th, it had been nearly four months since our last intimate moment. In fact, in the intervening weeks and months since the surgery, we hadn't done much of anything physical. Most of our good morning or goodbye kisses were on the cheek. Kirstin tried to kiss me in the hospital, but I pushed her away because I was worried about her reaction to kissing only half a functional mouth. She assured me that she was fine with it, but I was too ashamed and told her I wanted to wait until I was healed before we resumed intimacy. Days turned to weeks, which turned to months, and even now only 60% of my mouth works.

October 17th, 2015 was the fifty-two-week anniversary of our wedding (October 18th is the calendar anniversary) and we had not been intimate in nearly four months. Were there ever a time to force the romance, a wedding anniversary is the time. I got us reservations at one of her favorite restaurants and a hotel room at the hotel where we got married. There was champagne before dinner and chocolate cake afterward. She wore a floor-length purple dress and I wore a black suit and an eye patch. (Kirstin claims the eye patch is sexy, but I actually find them very uncomfortable and my eyeball gets hot and dry underneath). In any event, dinner was lovely and our parents (in cahoots with each other) arranged to pick up the tab. The night was going great.

When we got back to the hotel, we stopped in the hotel bar for a nightcap. After we charged the drinks to the room, we made our way to the elevator where we kissed passionately, but that would be the last cool move of my evening. When we got to the room, I searched my pants pocket for the key with my right hand with Kirstin holding my left. I couldn't find it. It was a real key, not a key card, with an enormous tassel on the end. How I lost it, I'm not sure, but it wasn't in my pants now and that left us standing out in the hallway. "It must have fallen out of my pocket," I said.

"You think!" Kirstin said with four months of exasperation on her face. "You stay here and I'll go find our key." As she walked back to the elevator, I was left standing outside the hotel room to ponder my stupidity.

Five minutes later, Kirstin returned with the room key, which had wedged itself in the couch where we were sitting. She brushed past me and opened the door quickly and deliberately. In the tiny hotel room, it only took three steps until we had arrived at the bed. I was nervous (and a little drunk), but I wanted this to be a special night, so I sat next to my wife in the bed and tried to be romantic. I kissed her gently on the neck, and after a few moments pressed her to the bed. In what I assumed would very a very dashing move, I put my arm across her body and rose so that my body was on top of hers. Unfortunately, my lack of general balance coupled with that last nightcap didn't allow me to stop my momentum, and I went rolling off the other side of the bed and quite inelegantly smacked my head on the nightstand.

"Are you okay?" Kirstin asked, looking down on me from the bed.

"Yes. I think I just fell on my pride," I joked, dabbing the back of my head to see if I was bleeding. She kissed my cheek and laughed. I laughed too. We spent the rest of the night icing my injuries and watching TV.

The next morning, we did resume our romantic endeavors, but this time without the head trauma.

OCTOBER AND NOVEMBER

The fall of 2015 was all about normalizing my life. I returned to work, attended a few Jets games with my father, but it wasn't normal. Every morning (within ten minutes of eating something) I would throw up. Most weekday afternoons, I would sneak in a nap in the school chaplain's office or at the nurse. Every night, within ten minutes of 8:00 p.m., I would lose the ability to walk with my own strength. The "8:00 p.m. rule" gradually became the "8:05 p.m. rule" and then the "8:10 p.m. rule" and so on, but it would be at least a year before I would comfortably allow myself out of the apartment after 10:00 p.m.

During the fall, I was weaned off certain medications and the morning sickness dissipated, but as much as I tried to normalize my life, I was still beholden to the recovery process. Twice a week, either before or after work, I would return to the hospital for physical therapy and occupational therapy in back-to-back sessions. These sessions were shorter and less frequent than when I was on the rehab floor, but the exercises were largely the same. It was a lot of toe tapping, balancing on one foot, sorting coins, and eye charts. Of course, I was supposed to do these exercises daily at home and of course, that didn't always happen. I'm someone who likes to work out, but even though these exercises had been shown to improve motor skills in patients with similar backgrounds to mine, the improvements were painfully incremental.

Because of health insurance requirements, certain "measurables" were assessed every four to six weeks. Those measurables were things like the amount of time it would take me to insert pegs into a board with my left hand. A second set of measurables tested my balance in different ways to determine my "fall risk." Other measurables tested grip strength, sensation, and the extent of my disconjugate gaze (which is measured in diopters).

The "nine-hole peg test" was simple enough: take nine wooden pegs the size of small screws and place them each into one of nine holes on a square wooden grid the size of a Sudoku puzzle from the newspaper. Then you take the nine pegs out of the grid and place them back on the table. When I did this task with my right hand it would generally take me about 30 seconds, but completing this task with my left hand presented many challenges. First, I could barely feel anything with my fingertips, so picking up small items was very difficult (and nearly impossible without looking). Second, I could not hold my arm or hand in one position for any discernible amount of time. In the fall of 2015, when I stretched my hand out in front of my body it would shake back and forth like a metronome by as much as six to eight inches in any direction. Usually the shaking receded after five or six seconds, but sometimes I would need to grab it with my right hand to get it to stop. Third, because I couldn't really feel my hand and because it would shake uncontrollably, I would often drop the pegs onto the table or the floor during the test. I cannot express how frustrating this assessment was for me in the fall of 2015, and it was on the menu nearly every OT session. In September of 2015, it took me two minutes and 45 seconds to complete the nine-hole peg test. Sadly, after two-plus months of practice, I was only down to two minutes and 34 seconds.

The second assessment I remember taking in mid-November was one to determine my fall risk. Certain measurements were taken, like the length of time I could stand on one leg or the ability to climb stairs, as well as the speed of my gait and ability to move laterally. Inability to complete certain tasks correlated with increased fall risk and the recommendation of certain types of assistance, such as a wheelchair or a shower stool. By the time I left the hospital, I had moved out of the wheelchair range and into the walker range. One month later, the assessment recommended the use of a cane only. By mid-November, despite my daily exercises and twice weekly visits to therapy, I was still assessed in the cane zone. (I still use a cane in public spaces, but walk freely at work and at home.)

The third test I remember taking in mid-November was to assess the degree of my disconjugate gaze. The test took two circles of different colors and placed them on separate transparencies, but on the same plane inside a backlit box. A person who had normal vision would only see the circles as one if they were placed on top of one another. A person with a disconjugate gaze would incorrectly fuse separate circles that were placed at a distance from one another. That distance is measured in units called prism diopters. Lower measurements of prism diopters can be fixed with prism glasses (less than 7). Higher measurements can often be fixed with surgery and prisms (less than 15). Anything higher than 15 cannot be fixed with surgery. I left the hospital with a prism diopter measurement around 28, and by mid-November I was only down to 24.

All of this is to say that after nearly five months of pretty intense therapy, while I had returned to work, could shower standing, and rode the train to work, the measurables of my disabilities due to the surgery had not changed in any significant way.

NEW YEAR'S EVE

New Year's Eve is perhaps my favorite holiday. Even though it's relatively arbitrary, the holiday marks the end of one thing and the beginning of another. It's true that there is often jockeying to find the best and biggest party, but it's also a celebration for the sake of celebrating and (in my opinion) an excellent opportunity to wear a tuxedo. For obvious reasons, I wanted to put 2015 behind me, and the new year happened to coincide with the sale of my in-laws' loft apartment of the previous 25 years. It might not sound like the coolest thing to throw parties at your in-laws' apartment, but this place was made for parties, and we were committed to sending it off with a bang. I floated this idea to Gary and Ingrid in mid-November, and once they agreed to let us host a party, I was so excited that I sent this email to my ten closest male friends:

> *Gentlemen,*
>
> *2015 was the worst year in the history of mankind! That is a scientific fact.*
>
> *If you don't have any plans already (and if you do you are a bigger nerd than me), please join Kirstin, me, and about seventy of our closest friends in saying "good riddance" to 2015 at Gary and Ingrid's Gramercy Penthouse.*
>
> *This will be the biggest, best, and last New Year's Eve party at 16th Street as Gary and Ingrid fly south for retirement.*
>
> *Cheers,*
>
> *"Titanium" Dan*
>
> *P.S. Who has two thumbs and a new avatar?*

There was an accompanying Paperless Post that was far more classy than what I had written above, but I think this email fully captures the irrational confidence I was trying to portray at that time. (P.S. "'Titanium' Dan" referenced the titanium mesh that was placed at the base of my skull to hold my head together. P.P.S. No, I don't set off metal detectors at airport security.) I was in denial and, by definition, I didn't know that I was in denial. In retrospect, what would come next should have been obvious, or at least was overdue; New Year's Eve would serve as the absolute low point in my recovery.

The in-laws' apartment was a 2500-square-foot loft-style apartment near Union Square. They purchased it in 1990, and now it was worth a lot more. The bedrooms were all clustered near the elevator, which opened directly into the apartment, and the vast majority of the domicile was open living space. Once you pushed the dining room table to the side, you got a pretty big dance floor and a space that could accommodate nearly 100 revelers. And at the party's peak, that was probably how many people were there. Kirstin had gotten a friend of a friend to DJ the event, and Kirstin's younger sister Elka, 25 at the time, accounted for most of the guests. Unfortunately for me, only one of the ten guys who got my mid-November invitation were able to attend, but we had all the makings of a good party and I was ready to leave 2015 in the past.

The day of the party was mostly taken up with preparation. Bags of ice were procured. Plastic cups were purchased. Party hats and those annoying New Year's Eve kazoos were placed around the apartment with care. Around 9:00 p.m., the DJ showed up with two large speakers, turntables, and crates of records. It was 2015, but whatever. Normally, I would offer to help carry the heavy items, but in my weakened state I contributed by manning the elevator. One would think in 2015, this would not be a necessity, but this apartment was in a converted factory and each floor needed to be unlocked with a key. It wasn't particularly exciting to man the elevator, but given that the downstairs buzzer was (yet again) not working, someone had to do it. Once the DJ was loaded in, I went to find Kirstin. She was in the bathroom with her sister and a few other women, primping and styling for the night. After standing awkwardly in the background with nothing to add to the conversation, I went into one of the bedrooms to change into my now very snug tuxedo. After ten minutes of sucking in my ever-expanding gut, I returned to the ladies' prep room and asked Kirstin to button my right sleeve (I didn't have the dexterity in my left hand to do it myself).

As she buttoned my sleeve, she said "Why don't you go hang out with the DJ? His name is Matt. He's a big sports guy as well. We're going to need a little bit more time in here." Getting the not-so-subtle hint, I left the bathroom and walked over to the living room where Matt was setting up his equipment. I meekly asked if I could get him anything.

He looked up from the array of wires, glancing at me in my ill-fitting tuxedo, eye patch, and cane, paused and said: "No, I'm good." I walked over to the bar area to see if I could help with the set-up there, but everything was all in order. I looked around the house, where Christmas lights had been hung and decorations placed, searching for something to do while we had no guests and my wife was busy getting ready. Just then I got a phone call from Kirstin's younger sister Elka asking me to let her in the building. She had forgotten her keys upstairs and Kirstin was not answering her phone.

"Hold on, I'll be right down." I still had the house and elevator keys in my pocket from earlier and raced down to get her. Raced was a bit of an exaggeration, because the elevator took forty seconds to make the ten-floor trip in one direction. After the elevator rose to the tenth floor and I rode it back down to the first floor, I opened the door for Elka and about seven of her friends.

"Thanks Dan, you're a lifesaver." The other party-goers also thanked me for letting them in, and with that I found my purpose. Once we made it to the top floor, I grabbed a glass of champagne and headed back to the elevator to shepherd people from the ground floor to the apartment. After each trip, I grabbed a new cup of champagne, eventually opting to simply travel up and down with a bottle. I probably went up and down another twenty times, mostly letting in people that I didn't know. I tried to alter my greeting every time a new set of guests arrived.

"Happy New Year, come on in."

"Welcome to New Year's, come on in."

"Welcome to the party."

"Happy Birthday."

I'm not quite sure what the revelers thought of the one-eyed slurring elevator operator, but I was having fun turning keys and pushing buttons. I probably didn't have twenty glasses of champagne if I provided twenty rides on the elevator, but in that hour and a half I drank enough champagne (probably Prosecco) to make a rhino dizzy. Kirstin found me after I got off the elevator the last time and said, "You're drunk."

"So, what if I am? Someone had to operate the elevator," I said, as if the one necessitated the other.

"I can't deal with you right now. This is supposed to be our party!" she fumed.

"You were doing your hair," I replied, feeling confident in my retort.

"Steve, can you do something about this?" my wife said, turning to one of my college buddies, who was eager to intervene.

"Sure. Let's go get some air," he said, pulling me back into the elevator for a short walk to the neighboring stoop in the cold city air. We sat there for a couple of minutes, talking about life and the things that had happened in the past six months. I don't remember the details as the world swayed before me, but I do remember feeling more alert when I noticed that it was 11:55, and I asked Steve to help get me back inside.

When we arrived at the tenth floor and entered the party, the thumping music, dimmed lights, and loud conversations wiped away whatever sobriety I thought I gained in the out-side air. "Let's go find Kirstin and dance," I said, pulling Steve, who was supporting me by my elbow, toward the middle of the party.

As we trudged through the crowd of people, someone poked me and said, "Cool eyepatch." In a different time, I would have taken it as a compliment, and I think it was meant as such, but on this night, it simply drew my attention to all that I wasn't.

We found Kirstin in the middle of the dance floor with a bunch of her friends. She snapped her judgmental right eyebrow in my direction: "Are you cool now?"

"Yes," I said. "I'm sorry." We kissed, a quick peck, and started dancing. Well, that's an overstatement. Kirstin was dan-cing, Steve was dancing, all the people around me were dancing. I was bobbing up and down without really moving my feet. As I got more comfortable, I started to the two-step side-to side dance that Will Smith tries to teach the guy from *King of Queens* in the movie *Hitch*. After the ball dropped, I started to loosen up a bit. I really got my blood flowing. I was sweating a little bit and walked off the dance floor to take off my jacket. Once, I had placed it on a chair and returned to the dance floor, I reached with my right hand to roll up my left sleeve. When that was done I reached down with my left hand to undo my right sleeve--to no avail. I stopped dancing and tried again. Nothing doing. I couldn't get a proper grip on the button. I tried and tried and tried. I was trying to be discrete when Kirstin came over and undid my sleeve button. All at once, it hit me.

"I can't do it. I can't undo the button." The music blared and the room was spinning. I was breathing heavily. "I can't undo the button. I can't undo the button." I kept repeating my-self over and over as tears started to stream down my face. I was panicking. The disability that I was trying to leave behind in 2015 was right there in 2016, and I was hyperventilating. I had convinced myself that one day, I'd wake up and all this would be behind me. One day, I'd be able to feel my left hand. One day, I'd be able to turn the page. All that disillusionment hit me in one champagne-infused moment when I couldn't undo my button. Steve and Kirstin rushed me off the dance floor and got me into bed. I was still mumbling, "I can't do it, I can't do it," as they got an ice pack and set up a bucket in case I got sick. Both Kirstin and Steve stayed with me until, out of sadness and exhaustion, I feel asleep. While I did not get sick that night, it was what I consider to be the absolute low point in my recovery.

But it was also the point where I started to accept my limitations and stopped dreaming that I would wake up the next day completely healed. I had built up this night in my head as a grand relaunch of my own personal well-being, but instead I gave everyone a very public look at how far I had fallen. It was one of the sadder moments of my life, but it was ultimately necessary for me to push forward to where I am today.

THE NEW YEAR AND HOW I GOT FAT

After the New Year's Eve debacle, I redoubled my efforts in the recovery process. I scheduled more time at the gym, more time with my therapist, and contacted a nutritionist. She gave me a lot of good advice, such as "don't eat fried foods" and "try to incorporate more vegetables into your diet," but when you can't move like you want to, you can't exercise like you want to, and you're only two months away from vomiting daily at the smell of bread, you are unlikely to have the willpower to eat a healthy and balanced diet. And I didn't.

It goes back to the first week after surgery where I literally didn't eat any solid foods. I lost 10 pounds in the week because of it, though undoubtedly much of my lost weight was leg muscle. In that first week, I had no appetite and everything that I ate tasted bland (a side effect of brain surgery in the brain stem). It was Howard that initially piqued my appetite with a pastrami sandwich, but that recklessly flowed into all kinds of salty/fried foods going forward. When the guys visited me in the hospital, they brought fried chicken the first time and pizza the second. My wife brought me hot dogs on July 4th and nearly every family member brought me pastries. With limited activities each day and nowhere to go, I devoured it all. By the time I left the hospital I had gained back all the weight I lost in the first week, plus ten more pounds. By the end of the summer I had gained ten more pounds, and by the end of the fall fifteen more.

On New Year's Day 2016, I weighed 210 pounds, thirty-five pounds more than what I weighed when I went into surgery and forty-five pounds more than my lowest weight. It was a long time coming, but before school started back up from winter break, I went to the store and bought pants that actually fit. I was no longer a 31-inch waist and it was time to admit that. I already knew this because I could no longer tuck in my work shirts. Well, that was the beginning. Toward the end of the fall semester, I couldn't even button my pants. I was holding my pants up by cinching a tight belt. Adding insult to fat injury, because my pants were the wrong size, the zipper would often come undone. I don't know if my zipper problems were common knowledge around the school, but I was constantly checking my "barn door" until, in January, I gave in and bought two new pairs of khakis with 36-inch waists. That was still not the right size for me and I had to inhale deeply to button them, but it was all I was willing to admit. As the store clerk watched my struggle to breathe in my new pants, I reassured him that "these pants are only temporary, so I don't want to go any bigger."

"That's what we all say," he responded in a bitchy tone before pivoting on his loafers and walking away with his 28-inch waist. Had he responded in a more sympathetic tone, he probably could have convinced me to purchase pants that actually fit, but I took his response as the insult that it was and used it as motivation to lose the surgery weight.

Despite my best efforts, I remaining in the 200-210 range throughout all of 2016 and most of 2017. Reeling from the aforementioned shopping experience, I survived nearly two full years on two pairs of pants. I wasn't the most fashionable of New Yorkers for those years, but truthfully, I never was anyway.

GOLDEN-EYE

The second phase in my conversion toward bionic man was the insertion of a "gold leaf" in my right eyelid on Friday, February 19th, 2016. This surgery was nearly eight months after the brain surgery and in retrospect should have been done months earlier. I hope people reading this can understand my reticence to going under the knife again, but this was a simple procedure by which a gold leaf, a small dot similar in size to those candy dots that come multicolored on a baking sheet, gets inserted into the eyelid. The purpose of this surgery was to help me blink my eyelid shut, because for the past eight months I had not been able to close my right eyelid on my own. Let me write that part again: *For eight months, I could not close my right eye without using my hands and a piece of tape.*

Eerily, but not surprisingly since my ophthalmologist was affiliated with the same hospital, Kirstin and I checked in for this surgery at almost the exact same location as the first surgery, just two floors down and two hours later in the day. Thankfully, once we checked in we didn't have to wait long for the surgeon to greet us.

"Good morning, Daniel," said the bubbly ophthalmologist.

"Good morning, Dr. Moss. This is my wife Kirstin."

"Nice to meet you," he said with a smile.

"You can't take ten hours this time, doc," she quipped while squeezing my hand nervously.

"Oh no," he responded. "This is a simple procedure. You should be on your way home by noon at the latest." It was 8:00 a.m. at the time.

He turned to me. "Now, Daniel, I'm going to place a few stickers on your eyelid, and we'll see which one gives you the best ability to close your eyelid without having it droop down too much in the relaxed state." He reached forward and with his finger gently pulled down my right eyelid and placed a relatively small sticker on its exterior. "Okay, now open your eye and try to close it again."

"Holy shit," I exclaimed, blinking my eye for the first time in eight months. It was like touching the ocean for the first time, but without the salt and only with your eyeball. The closing of the eye is the body's natural way to keep the eye hydrated and wipe away dirt and other particles. For eight months, I had been manually closing my eyelid with my finger, applying eye drops ten times a day, and taping it shut at bedtime. With the placement of a sticker, I was able to close my eye simply by thinking about it. It was difficult and it didn't (and doesn't) move in perfect concert with the left eye, but if I think about blinking my right eye, I can do it. It was a magic in the form of a sticker.

"Holy shit," I said one more time.

"Okay," the doctor responded, "I think that one is a little too heavy. Do you see how his eyelid is drooping?" he asked in the direction of my wife. She nodded in accord. "Let's try a slightly lighter version," he said, reaching toward my eye. I wanted to stop him and say, *screw the surgery, just give me the stickers,* but I didn't. He removed the first and placed a lighter sticker in its place. I blinked a few times and looked toward my wife. "Better" he said, and asked my wife, who nodded in agreement. He tried one more before settling on the second sticker as the winner.

"Okay, I think we have the right weight for the insert. I'm going to head back and scrub in, and a nurse should come to get you in a few minutes." He smiled, shook my hand and then Kirstin's, and was gone.

"Sounds easy enough," I said, turning to my wife.

"I don't want you to go," she said, tearing up as much because of the memory of the last surgery as because of nervousness for this one.

"He said it's a pretty simple surgery and that we should be done in a few hours. I'll be fine," I said, trying to reassure her. But I had only been in the operating room; I had never been the one waiting on the other side. The last surgery was supposed to take five hours and it took ten. The last surgery was supposed to require seven days of recovery, but it took twenty. A lot of me was lost in that first surgery and I understand why this one brought up emotions for Kirstin, but this surgery was more about putting me back together than taking me apart.

We hugged for a few minutes and then a nurse pulled back the curtain to my patient cubicle, signaling that it was time for Kirstin to go. "Love you," she said before kissing me and retreating behind the curtain. "Don't take too long," she said to the nurse as she walked away.

The nurse gave a half-smile, acknowledging, but not understanding Kirstin's request before turning to me. "Are you ready, Mr. Rufer?" I nodded and started to rise when she responded: "Oh no, Mr. Rufer, you just stay in the chair and I'll wheel you in." Why the hospital would wheel you in for a simple procedure and make you walk into brain surgery is beyond me, but I sat back for the ride as we wheeled past the waiting room, made what seemed like seventy-five turns, and passed through forty-two sets of swinging double doors before arriving at the surgical suite.

This operating room was much smaller than the one from eight months ago. It was probably fifteen feet by twenty feet. I don't remember much about it because there wasn't much to remember. It was quite barren and felt much like a dental exam room had been expanded to twice its normal size. Everything was on rollable carts, from the surgical instruments (none of which I could see) to the lights to the IV bags. One thing I do remember is that it was extremely cold in this operating room. The nurse who had wheeled me in exited the room shortly after arrival, but returned with an electric blanket. I was starting to feel cozy in this barren and sterile environment.

Then in walked a hulking man wearing scrubs and a Yankees bandana tied around his head. He would soon reveal himself to be the anesthesiologist. I've now had six surgeries and I think every anesthesiologist that was assigned to me moonlighted as a bouncer in their spare time. Perhaps the extra muscle comes in handy should they have to ever hold someone down. In any event, he introduced himself without shaking my hand or even looking up from his chart. We reviewed my medical history and he made some notes, presumably about the dosage for the anesthesia. This time, I wouldn't be going completely under, but I would be heavily sedated for the surgery.

"Do you have any questions for me?" the anesthesiologist asked, looking up to meet my gaze for the first time.

"I'm a Mets fan," I stated. "Do you feel that you will be able to give me adequate consideration given the fact that my team was in the World Series last year and yours did not make the playoffs?"

In another environment, I'm sure we could have bonded over such playful ribbing. Instead, he responded: "I'll take that as a no," before turning to leave the room. "A surgical nurse will be in shortly to start you on an IV."

I turned to the nurse that brought me down. "He's not much of people person, is he?" She shrugged and we waited a few minutes in silence for the surgical nurse. Without much wasted time, she popped an IV in my arm and I feel asleep.

I awoke to find myself lying down, but on the same chair on which I was transported (it folded out into a bed apparently). I could hear three or four people talking in the room and could feel light pressure and heat on my right eyelid. The operation was underway and even though I was awake and very calm, my limbs felt pleasantly heavy and the anesthesia took away the desire to wiggle or move.

"Dr. Moss?" I asked.

"Yes?" he said, a detached voice above my head.

"How are you?" I slurred.

"I'm good, Daniel. We've started the surgical process so it's important that you stay still."

"Okay." I paused. "Did you see the anesthesiologist? What a jerk. I mean, I was only joking about the Yankees. I mean, it's not every year that we make it to the World Series. We have a good team..." I rambled on for a little while longer before a deep authoritative voice interrupted.

"Mr. Rufer." It was the anesthesiologist. "If you don't stop talking right now, I'm going to have to put you under."

"*Sooooo-reey,*" I said, like a child being reprimanded for stealing a cookie. "Hey Yankee fan, are you Jets or Giants?"

Dr. Moss chimed in: "Daniel, I really need you to be still for this part."

"Sorry." This time I was sincere. I remained quiet for the rest of the surgery and, true to his word, Dr. Moss had me in a taxi on my way home by noon. The surgery gave me a pretty gnarly black/green/purple eye, but after a week or so, the swelling had receded and I was able to close my right eye just by thinking about it. Given the myriad other problems I was dealing with, fixing my eyelids seemed relatively minor at the time, but being able to sleep without tape on my eye and reducing my eyedrop intake from 10 times a day to three was a huge boon to my confidence and morale. Cosmetically, I no longer looked like a guppy on the right side of my face, and it signaled a new stage of the recovery process.

SLEEP, THAT'S WHERE I'M A VIKING

It's been said that the subconscious mind reveals the truest form of one's self. If we are to take dreams at face-value, I am a world-class wide receiver, a dominating power hitter, and a very handsome secret agent. Though I am pushing forty, my dreams are still often related to sports accolades. Interestingly, despite the last eight months (now, at the time of publication, three years) I am never disabled in my dreams. I'm still catching Super Bowl-winning touchdowns, hitting towering home runs, and executing windmill dunks in the NBA finals. Since I can't control my subconscious, I can't tell you why I still dream about sports like an adolescent boy, but I do. I think having a playful subconscious is a big part of what made me a good middle school teacher. It may have held me back in adult relationships, but I think it helps me relate to children because (on a subconscious level) I never really grew up.

At some point in mid-March 2016, I was having a dream in which I was playing wide receiver for the Jets in the Super Bowl. (Insert Jets joke here.) Anyway, like many dreams, it was not particularly linear in nature. I do know that in the dream, we were down four with ten seconds left to go in the game when I gave a knowing look to an anonymous quarterback that he should throw the ball my way. I was lined up wide on the left side facing one-on-one coverage. At the snap I took three quick steps to the inside as the quarterback executed a pump-fake and I broke in the opposite direction. The quarterback delivered a lofting jump-ball to the leftmost corner of the end zone. It hung in the air for what seemed like an eternity and was slightly behind my route. At the last moment I reached up with my left hand and plucked the ball out of the air, securing the pass, the touchdown, and the championship.

"What the fuck is wrong with you?" screamed my wife while punching me in the gut.

I sat up quickly, and sadly realized that I was not a Super Bowl-winning wide receiver. I had not made the greatest catch in NFL history. I was a man in bed with his wife whose subconscious had mistakenly led him to punch her in the face. I was sleeping on my back, as I typically do, and when the subconscious Daniel reached out to catch the pass, the sleeping Daniel recklessly extended his left arm, making immediate and startling contact with his wife's face below the right eye.

"What the hell are you doing?" she asked, reaching to turn on the light on her nightstand.

As I tried to catch my bearings, I said "I'm sorry, babe, I was dreaming and I must have hit you by mistake."

"You were dreaming?"

"Yes, well I wasn't dreaming of hitting you. In my dream I was a receiver in the Super Bowl and I was trying to--"

"You know what, I don't give a shit. Please don't hit me in the face."

"Got it. Roger that. I'm sorry. Do you want me to get you some ice?"

"No, it'll be okay, just try not to hit me in your sleep."

"Yes, of course," I said as she turned off the light and turned away from me, assuming a protective curled position. As I sat up in bed I thought about the absurdity of me making a one-handed catch with my (disabled) left arm. That was not a realistic catch for me to make with my right hand as a teenager, yet my mind dreamt I could do it and my body followed with a similar movement in real life. I was certainly sorry to have smacked my wife in the face while she was sleeping, but it comforted me to know that my subconscious hadn't given up hope of an able-bodied life.

Maybe it was time for my conscious body to play catch-up.

A CONVERSATION WITH THE GOOD REVEREND

Why didn't I die?

It's a question I often thought about. Were I born at any point before 1970 (and that's being conservative) the technology to detect and identify cavernous malformations (MRI machines) would not have been available, and had mine continue to bleed I most certainly would have died. Had I been born after 1970 but diagnosed before 2000, the surgical techniques would have been more invasive and I might have died. Had I waited another week, the malformation could have bled more and I could have died. The surgery itself was estimated for five hours, but took nearly ten and I could have died. There were so many ways in which the cavernous malformation could have been fatal, and yet through a confluence of fate and modern science, I didn't die. Why?

Eventually I was able to settle on the most obvious reason why I didn't die: the surgery saved my life. Yet that comfort was short-lived as another, more philosophical question replaced my unknowing: *should I be dead?*

It's such a deep question that even though I was going to talk therapy once a week, unpacking my feelings/anger/sadness about my slow recovery, we never pivoted to discuss my feelings about simply being alive. For that conversation, I sought out the person whom I thought would have the most experience pondering existence: our school Chaplin, the good Reverend Hummell.

I didn't know how long this conversation would take, nor how emotional it would be, so rather than meeting during lunch or in between classes at school, we decided to meet at his apartment in upper Manhattan over spring break. It was a Tuesday and I remember the walk from the train station that day because though it was sunny and unusually warm for mid-March, the cool breeze coming off the Hudson both chilled my bones and made it difficult to climb the slope toward Riverside Drive. I remember feeling disoriented once I was in the building lobby because I no longer had to counteract the force of the wind and my inner ear was still telling me to lean forward. Without the breeze, my core immediately warmed, and I pushed the button in the elevator for the sixth floor.

When I exited the elevator and turned left to find his lettered apartment. He was standing in the doorway. "Welcome to Washington Heights," he said, stepping aside to reveal a living room with couches facing large windows overlooking the George Washington Bridge, the Hudson River, and the Palisades mountain range. It was a calming and pristine view on this warm spring day. "Can I get you anything to drink? Water? Iced tea?"

"Water would be great," I responded, taking a moment to size up the apartment just as any born-and-bred New Yorker would. When he returned from the kitchen I pivoted away from the window and took a seat on the couch. He sat on an adjacent chair to my left.

"You indicated over email that you wanted to have a philosophical conversation. What did you have in mind?"

"Well, I don't know exactly how to phrase this." I paused to search for the right words. "I guess what I'm trying to figure out... what I'm not understanding about my illness is why I'm still alive."

"Oh, that is a big question," he responded before pausing for a couple of seconds and shifting in his seat. "Well, why do you think you're alive?"

"C'mon, Rev. If I wanted that kind of response I could have posted my question on the internet."

He half-laughed and said, "No, I guess what I mean to say is that it doesn't matter why I think you are alive--why do you think you are alive? Conversely, why do you think this illness happened in the first place?"

"Well" I responded, feeling as if I could engage in this line of questioning a bit more. "I don't know why it happened to me. The research I did on the topic just says that cavernous malformations tend to occur to men in their thirties, but are extremely rare and might be hereditary. And when they do occur, they can occur anywhere in the brain and can cause a myriad of symptoms or no symptoms at all. It's quite possible I have had the cav-mal my entire life, but it only started expressing symptoms a year ago. I guess the long and the short of it is that this feels totally random and I don't get why it happened to me."

Reverend Hummel pushed back. "I don't think you totally believe that. That anyone could have this illness or that it exists might be completely random, but why did *you* get this illness and not someone else? If you were a member of the church, I might ask why you thought God chose you to carry this burden."

I'm not sure if I believe in God. I believe in the existence of something higher than man, but not necessarily God, or a God, or the Christian God per se. I am a math teacher and believe in the order and measure of the universe, but some things can't be explained by equations or vectors. And that's what troubled me about this illness. Were I a smoker and got lung cancer, science has told us that there is a high probability that the smoking caused the cancer. Were I an avid sun-bather and got skin cancer, science has told us that there is a high probability that the tanning caused the cancer. But in this case, in my case, the science told us next to nothing, or at the very least it has told us very little thus far. Why I had a cavernous malformation and my father doesn't is unknown. Or more confusingly, maybe he does, but it doesn't act up in the same way. Some things, and this was one of them, appeared random and terrible. And that was unsettling, because if my illness was a random act, then so was meeting my wife, or finding my job, or being born at all. When you extrapolate out from a random event, it leaves you in a very uncomfortable place. This didn't feel random to me. It wasn't flipping a coin or rolling the dice. This was my life, and I was uncomfortable thinking it was completely random.

After a few moments of thinking, I said, "I think I have this illness because on some level I can handle it. It may sound narcissistic, but in a weird way, I was built to have this experience. I was essentially born at the right time to have this diagnosed in this exact way. Were I born fifty years ago, it would have never been discovered. In fifty years, maybe there will be a pill to cure cavernous malformations. Who knows? But for right now, at this moment in time, I was built for this. I live in the city with the best hospitals in the world. I have a career that I can still maintain even after being crippled by the surgery. I have a wife that loves me and cares for me. I can't imagine being single and going through this." I paused, starting to tear up. Rev passed me a tissue, then leaned back in his chair to let me continue talking. "If I was younger, I don't think I would have agreed to the surgery. If I was older, the recovery would have been nearly impossible. If I was heavier, there is no way those tiny therapists in the hospital could have moved me. Being thirty-four, weighing the least I ever weighed as an adult because of a ridiculous wedding regime, and being married were all factors that allowed me to come through this experience and be here today."

"See?" the good reverend said, and smiled. "That doesn't sound random at all."

We continued to talk for another half hour about the fickle nature of health and how finding one's place in the world can often feel like a journey of random events. But what I came to understand from that conversation and what I still truly believe is that when you find that place where you are supposed to be, all those random events do serve some purpose. These events do start to make sense. I still don't understand why all this happened to me, and honestly, I don't care. But, what I truly believe is that all this happened to me because that's what was meant to happen. As I write this paragraph even I'm rolling my eyes, but I never wonder *why me* anymore? And I never wonder why I didn't die. I simply cherish the fact that I am here with the woman that I love, doing a job that I love, and pushing myself to get better every day.

DON'T CALL IT A COMEBACK

Thursday, May 26th was the day before the first-ever high school graduation ceremony at Grace Church School. But, more importantly, it was the opening game in the 2016 Flying Squirrels' softball season. I had previously told the players on my team that I would manage them for the season, but on the walk over to the field I decided I would take one at-bat. This game was scheduled at the normally undesirable East River field, but since I was coming from work, it was actually the easiest field for me to get to on this particular day.

At about 5:00 p.m., I left my office in full squirrel uniform. I wore my Flying Squirrel t-shirt jersey, aqua-blue mesh shorts, a bright red knee-high sock on my left leg only, black ankle brace, grey sneakers, and backwards fitted blue Mets hat. It was not an ensemble designed by professionals, but I like to think that the mismatched outfit helped lull the other team into a sense of superiority regarding their matching clothing. Anyway, I called for a car that let me out on the west side of FDR Drive and Houston Street. I put on my backpack full of math tests as I exited the car and extended my cane to start my journey over the highway and down to the field. Butterflies filled my stomach as a combination of nerves and hot, humid weather weighed on my shoulders. As I walked down the ramp from the overpass and through the metal gating that surrounded the field, I was greeted by a bunch of my teammates who were finishing warming up for the season's first competition.

Even though I was limping heavily, walking with a cane,

and winded from a 500-foot journey from the other side of the highway, I was greeted with smiles and positive salutations.

"Hey Rufer. Welcome back."

"You look great"

"Good to see you."

And then from my buddy Dave: "Are you playing?"

"I'll take one at-bat at some point during the game, but I'm not playing the field."

"Obviously, but are you sure that's a good idea?"

"Dave," I paused and put an arm around his shoulder. "I almost died a year ago. I'm taking a fucking at-bat." He had no argument for that. And so, I sloppily sunk into the turf and began stretching my bum leg.

After about five minutes, I was called to home plate to hear the ground rules. The umpire was a man named Angel whom I had known for ten years. "It's good to see you back, Dan," he said before explaining the ground rules of the field, which had not changed in the twenty-five years since I played Little League on this very spot. I took in the view while he talked and then returned to my team.

"Okay, bring it in!" I yelled while limping to the first base dugout where we were stationed. Once everyone was huddled up, I asked for a slow clap while I read out the line-up.

"Leading off as the DH is me. Batting second and playing second is Karen, batting third and in left field is Eric...." When I finished the line-up, I looked around the huddle of confused faces and said, "Relax people. If I get on, I'll take a runner." That did not seem to ease the tension. "Look, I make the line-up and I almost died, so I'm batting first." Some smiles and laughter broke through the nervous glances. "Okay, here we go." I paused before yelling "One-Two-Three, Squirrels!" to which my teammates responded:

"Go nuts!"

I borrowed a batting glove from Eric as I walked up to the batter's box using the bat as a cane. I had no idea how this was going to go, but I was damned if I wasn't going to try to resume a normal life. I stepped into the batter's box on the left side of home plate and instinctively tapped the dirt off my sneakers even though the field was entirely turf and it was completely unnecessary. Angel asked if I was ready. Once I nodded and pulled my sunglasses over my eyes, he squatted back and said, "Play ball."

This was co-ed slow-pitch high-arc softball, so I wasn't particularly worried about catching up to the speed of the pitch. However, I was very concerned with two things. First, I was concerned that I wouldn't be able to hit the ball because of a lack of depth perception; I had taped over the right lens on the inside of all my sunglasses to avoid my double-vision. Secondly, I was concerned that I wouldn't be able to hold onto the bat through the swing. I thought there was a distinct possibility that as I swung the bat through the zone, the bat would go flying, and that I would be charged with murdering the pitcher or shortstop. The first was a worry of vanity, the second was a worry of legality. I tried to put those concerns out of my mind as I watched the first pitch land directly behind home plate for strike one. Ever since high school, I always took the first pitch to get a sense of the pitcher. It was probably unnecessary in softball, but considering this was my first at-bat in nearly two years, I think it was an apt strategy. I had followed the ball all the way to the ground and convinced myself that I could do this. As the next pitch came in, slowly reaching its apex at about twelve feet and breaking to chest height over the plate, I squeezed the bat as hard as I could with my left hand and swung the bat through the zone. Without even feeling it, I had struck a line drive over the pitcher's head. I had (and still have) trouble picking up fast-moving things in my field of vision, so I didn't see the ball until it was already past second base and in the outfield. It was at that moment that I realized I had to run to first base. I pivoted away from the outfield and sent signals from my brain to my legs that we had to run. I looked like Road Runner skidding in place before take-off as my right leg compiled and my left leg dragged behind. Before I could get my left leg out in front of me, I fell to the ground. The ball was already in the center fielder's glove. With my teammates both cheering and laughing, I got up and limp-ran to first base, barely beating a throw from the outfield before collapsing five feet behind the bag in exhaustion. (See www.disconjugategaze.com for footage).

As I lay on my back trying to catch my breath, I looked up at the clear sky, reflecting on all that had happened in the past year. That was as ugly a hit as you are ever going to see, but in that moment, I proved to myself that I was capable of anything. Well, not literally anything, but certainly more than most would assume were they watching me limp from the car to the field. After a few seconds I rolled over onto my right side, picked myself up, and walked to first base before calling for a runner and accepting the high fives from my teammates.

"Tell me you got that on video?" I asked, panting.

"Yep," Joanna said before passing my phone back to me. As I sat on the bench watching the video of my first at-bat in two years, pride swelled in my chest. Because I don't do social media, I forwarded the video to my wife, parents, cousins, and about five other friends with the tag line "Don't call it a comeback." (Shout-out to LL Cool J.)

I shockingly went 3 out of 4 that game and batted .500 for the season. To be fair, that was about 150 points below my normal summer softball league average, but not bad for someone with one functioning leg, one functioning eye, and numbness in his lead hand. I played DH in all ten games that season before retiring at the end of the season. In retrospect, it probably was not wise to play softball that summer. Had I rolled an ankle or twisted my knee I would have seriously endangered the recovery process. But as someone who played sports his entire life and feels most at ease on the athletic field, I chose to define myself not by what I couldn't do, but by what I could.

CLOSING EXERCISES

When you go through a life-altering experience, there are a lot of milestones that are emotional along the way. Most of them are firsts, like the first time I walked without a cane, or the first time I hit a softball. Others remind you of the way things were. The high school closing exercises on Tuesday, June 14th was like that for me. A year prior, when I addressed the Class of 2018, I did it wondering if it was going to be the last time any of them would ever see me. I knew I was having surgery and I knew that I might die, but I didn't tell any of them. I savored every summer goodbye because I knew it might be my last. I was holding in the secret because I am a reserved person, but also because the closing exercises are about the students and there was no need to take away from their day. A year later, very much alive, but very different in profound ways, I addressed the Class of 2018 as I bid them farewell for the summer:

> This self-reflection is written with the vocabulary and temperament of a sophomore in high school, but delivered by a thirty-something-year-old mediocre orator.
>
> Overall, I think I did a pretty good job in my second year as a dean at Grace Church High School. Despite a literal hole in my head, I only missed four work days (one due to illness, one to unnavigable snow, and two personal days). With the help of an amazing advising team, I think I planned a pretty fun scavenger hunt to kick off sophomore year, though ordering ice cream sandwiches on a 90-degree September day was not my best decision.

One thing I would like to improve upon is in relation to my hair. It has been a difficult transition for me away from youthful locks to middle-age thinning. I could really use some help, advice, and support in the area of hair styling over these next two years.

One thing I would like to highlight is my continued ability to snipe gum-chewers. Even with one functioning eyeball, I feel I have successfully curbed the gum-chewing inclinations of the Class of 2018. Next year, I plan to mount an assault on dangling earbuds in the hallway. I think I can find a way to prosecute offenders under the New York State fire code, but I will have to talk to our friends in Albany before unveiling a new attack strategy.

In terms of the way I feel, I am (mostly) proud of the Class of 2018. You pushed me to churn out behavioral alerts at break-neck speed this past marking period, but you also accomplished a lot this year. For example, you completed March Madness, the history research paper, and blank space to be filled before speech for standard three example speech-reading trinity of examples. Yes, we stumbled along the way. Some of us even stumbled into a desk with our heads. But we are now through a year of tremendous change and growth. Now, all you have to do is take the SATs, fill out college applications, write several more research papers, possibly learn to drive, convince me to attend prom, and actually go to your PE classes, Like, literally!

Are the next two years going to be difficult and stressful? Yes, very. But the next two years will push your limits and you will come out the other side better equipped to handle change, better at managing your time & stress, and hopefully (with a little prodding from your advisors) better as a team.

ON A PLANE

The last chapter of this book is not the end of my recovery. That is an ongoing and lifelong journey. The last chapter in this book ends the twelve-month saga of surgery and recuperation on nearly the exact day when my wife and I were supposed to go on our honeymoon. On October 18th, 2014, Kirstin and I pledged ourselves to each other for better or worse and in sickness and in health. Little did we know that those famous vows would be put to the test a little more than six months later or that our honeymoon, so carefully planned, would be cancelled, and that instead of two weeks in Italy, we would spend three weeks in a hospital. It was an unfair trade, one that no person in their right mind would make, but ultimately, we didn't have a choice. Thankfully, I had someone who pledged themselves to me and with whom I was able to navigate this unwanted journey.

Our honeymoon, postponed indefinitely in 2015, was rescheduled in 2016. We decided that while Italy was beautiful, going there and trying to do all the things that we had planned in 2015 would be too emotionally painful. After months of back-and-forth, we decided to go on an African safari. We are very blessed to be able to afford such a vacation, and Africa presented itself as the perfect opposite to a vacation in Italy. In Italy, food is the attraction. In Africa, the attractions can eat you.

On July 3rd, 2016, Kirstin and I set off on the honeymoon that we didn't get in 2015. We had a send-off party and safari gear fashion show with our friends before we left. Our friend Adam drove us to Newark International Airport where we checked our bags and tried to put the past twelve months behind us. Being disabled sucks, but being disabled in an airport is pretty great. We were whisked through TSA and were the first to board the sixteen-hour flight to Arusha, Tanzania. I let Kirstin take the window seat and sat in the middle. We rearranged our stuff in the seat-back pockets while everyone else boarded the plane. After the emergency instructions were read and the plane taxied to the designated runway, I tapped Kirstin for attention while she looked out the window.

When she turned to me, I grabbed her right hand in my left and asked "You ready?" She smiled in response and squeezed my left hand as the plane accelerated and zipped down the runway before rising and taking flight into the summer sky.

ACKNOWLEDGEMENTS

Forgive my redundancy, but I'd first like to thank my wife for supporting and loving me throughout this process and for forcing me to keep the "accomplishments journal" that became the basis for this book.

Second, I'd like to thank my parents, sister, and in-laws for supporting Kirstin and myself when times were the most tough. Similarly, I'd like you thank all the friends who came to visit me in the hospital. Though the visits were exhausting, they broke up the monotony of therapy and kept me sane.

Third, I'd like to thank Liza Birnbaum, my editor extraordinaire, who saw typos and verb disagreement where I saw none. Though we have never met in person, I have enjoyed our phone conversations and electronic correspondence these past six months. And, I'd like to thank Brian Platzer for introducing me to Liza and guiding me through the writing process. This would not have been possible without your counsel.

Fourth, I'd like to thank all the health care professionals: Dr. Ross, Dr. Adams, Kimberly, and the rest of in-hospital team. Your kindness will never be forgotten. I'd also like to thank my post-surgery recovery team of positive energy folks: Amy Fitzpatrick (acupuncture), Casey Leigh Carty (acupuncture), and Jason Maggard (physical therapy).

Fifth, I'd like to thank Chandra Claypool for her publishing and marketing advice and Elka Bunton for showing me how to operate the Facebook and the Twitter and the Instagram.

Lastly, I'd like to thank the faculty, administration, families, and children of Grace Church School. In the fall of 2015, you received me with love and smiles that I really needed at that time. Despite my physical deficiencies, I have never felt "less than" when I'm at Grace.

Super-lastly, I'd like to thank you, the reader of this book. I hope my story provides you with some insight as to the impact a health crisis can have on individuals, families, and friends. I hope this book also underscores that while life isn't always easy, if you try to put one foot in front of the other, eventually you'll get somewhere.

ABOUT THE AUTHOR

I am a Mathematics Teacher and Grade Dean in the High School Division at Grace Church School in downtown Manhattan. I am a lifelong New Yorker as is my wife Kirstin. We have been married for almost four years and together for slightly more than ten. We live together with our dog, Moxie, in Long Island City.

My undergraduate degree is in Economics from Vassar College and I hold master's degrees in Teaching Mathematics and Educational Leadership from City College and N.Y.U respectively. I am a long-suffering Mets, Jets, and Knicks fan, but believe that championships will come before the end of the 21st Century.

Made in the USA
Middletown, DE
17 December 2019

80962188R00099